Mary A.Clapp

SIMONE BILES

Mary A.Clapp

"BREAKING BARRIERS: HOW SIMONE BILES BECAME A GYMNASTICS LEGEND"

Mary A.Clapp

Mary A.Clapp

Mary A. Clapp

Mary A.Clapp

TABLE OF CONTENTS

Mary A.Clapp

Mary A.Clapp

Mary A.Clapp

Mary A.Clapp

Mary A.Clapp

WHO IS SIMONE BILES?

One of the most talented artistic gymnasts of all time, Simone Biles is an American gymnast of exceptional skill. Here is a summary of her life and accomplishments:

Childhood Date of Birth: On March 14, 1997, Simone Arianne Biles was born in Columbus, Ohio.

Household: Because of their mother's issues with substance misuse, she and her sister were adopted by Ron and Nellie Biles, who raised her.

Gymnastics Discovery: When Biles was six years old, she went on a field trip from her daycare and found gymnastics. She soon started training. She advanced fast because it was clear from the beginning that she had talent.

Mary A.Clapp

CAREER IN GYMNASTICS

Young Professional: When Biles started competing nationally in 2011, her strong routines and high difficulty level helped her establish a reputation for herself.

High School Debut: In 2013, she participated in her first senior international competition and took home the all-around title in the World Championship.

OLYMPIC ACCOMPLISHMENTS RIO OLYMPICS 2016

Gold Medals: Floor Exercise, Vault, Team, and All-Around Balance Beam (Bronze Medal)- Biles became an overnight sensation at the Rio Olympics, taking home more gold medals in the women's gymnastics competition than any other American in history.

Tokyo Olympics 2020 (held in 2021): Team Event: Silver Medal- Balance Beam (Bronze Medal)- Biles struggled with mental health issues throughout these

Mary A.Clapp

Olympics, which included having "the twisties," a perilous illness that impairs a gymnast's sense of spatial awareness.

 With 25 medals, including 19 gold, as of 2024, Biles is the most decorated gymnast in the history of the World Championships. She has given the sport various new talents that bear her name, including:

The Biles on Floor Exercise: This is a half-out double arrangement.

The Biles on Vault: A double pike by Yurchenko.

The Biles on Balance Beam: A double backflip dismount that twists twice.

INFLUENCE AND ADVOCACY

Advocacy for Mental Health: Biles has made a strong case for the value of mental health, particularly in light of her experiences competing in the Tokyo Olympics. Her candor has motivated a lot of people and raised

Mary A.Clapp

awareness of the challenges encountered by professional athletes.

Survivor Perspectives: She testified against former USA gymnastics doctor Larry Nassar and has been a champion for survivors of sexual assault in gymnastics.

Party Model: For young athletes, especially women of color, Biles is blazing a path in fields that have historically been controlled by others.

Latest Advancements Return: In 2023, Simone Biles returned to competition with success, breaking records and carrying on her legacy by earning her eighth national all-around title at the U.S. Gymnastics Championships.

Intimate Life: In February 2022, Biles revealed her engagement to NFL player Jonathan Owens; the two were married in 2023.

LEGACY

Mary A.Clapp

 Result: By elevating the standard for athleticism and artistry and inspiring the next generation of gymnasts, Simone Biles has had a huge impact on the sport of gymnastics.

Identification: Due to her achievements in sports and society, she has been recognised as one of Time magazine's "100 Most Influential People" and has won other accolades. Simone Biles' remarkable talent, tenacity, and activism are demonstrated by her rise from a young gymnast to an international celebrity.

Her experience and commitment to mental health and athlete safety have inspired individuals all across the world, and her influence goes beyond gymnastics. One of the most talented artistic gymnasts of all time, Simone Biles is an American gymnast of exceptional skill. Here is a summary of her life and accomplishments:

Mary A.Clapp

INTRODUCTION

Very few athletes in the world of sports become great icons. With her unmatched achievements and innovative energy, Simone Biles has not only transformed gymnastics but also gone beyond athletic bounds to become a symbol of activism, resiliency, and empowerment. This book explores Simone Biles's multifarious influence on gymnastics and beyond by going inside her path, her struggles, her victories, and the enduring legacy she leaves behind.

The Revolution of Gymnastics The influence of Simone Biles on gymnastics is significant and varied. Recognised for her exceptional strength, dexterity, and technical accuracy, Biles has raised the bar for performance in the sport. She has created brand-new, eponymous feats that exhibit a level of difficulty never seen in gymnastics before. She has broken records, won multiple world titles, and won over admirers all over the world with her performances.

This book will examine how a new generation of athletes has been motivated and how the limits of gymnastics have been redefined by Biles' ground-breaking performances.

Individual Difficulties and Successes Beyond her physical ability, Simone Biles has exhibited incredible fortitude in the face of adversity. Her narrative is one of bravery and resolve as she navigates the intense constraints of elite competition and overcomes obstacles in her early life. Important discussions regarding athlete well-being and the significance of mental health support in sports have been spurred by Biles' candor about her issues with mental health, especially during the Tokyo 2020 Olympics. This book will look at how her openness has inspired others to give mental health first priority and get help when they need it.

Empowerment and Advocacy Beyond gymnastics, Simone Biles has advocated for positive change through her platform. She has been a strong voice for victims of sexual assault, opposing former USA gymnastics physician Larry Nassar and calling for transparency in the industry. Through her advocacy work, Biles has brought attention to the structural problems with gymnastics and sparked significant changes meant to protect athletes. Numerous people have been inspired to tell their tales and seek justice by her bravery in speaking out.

Motivating Next Generations Simone Biles has torn down boundaries and dispelled preconceptions in the gymnastics industry, which has historically been dominated by women of color. Her accomplishments have served as an inspiration to young athletes around the globe, proving that everything is achievable with hard work, enthusiasm, and determination.

This book will examine how Biles' influence goes well beyond her accomplishments and continues to inspire and motivate upcoming generations of athletes and gymnasts from all backgrounds. The goal of "Breaking Barriers: How Simone Biles Became a Gymnastics

Mary A.Clapp

Legend" is to distill the remarkable journey of Simone Biles to its core.

This book strives to honor a unique athlete who has changed gymnastics and inspired countless people worldwide through an in-depth examination of her impact on the sport, advocacy efforts, and personal victories. The life of Simone Biles is one of tenacity, fortitude, and the eternal strength of the human spirit; her legacy will serve as an inspiration to future generations.

CHAPTER 1: EARLY LIFE AND BEGINNINGS

On March 14, 1997, Simone Arianne Biles was born in Columbus, Ohio. Significant obstacles in her early childhood laid the groundwork for her eventual resilience and determination. Shanon Biles, a single mother battling addiction, gave birth to Simone, the third of her four siblings.

Mary A.Clapp

At the age of three, Simone and her siblings were placed in foster care as a result of these circumstances. In order to provide Simone with a secure environment, Ron Biles, her maternal grandpa, and his wife Nellie Cayetano Biles intervened in 2000. Their great-aunt adopted their other siblings, but they formally adopted Simone and Adria, her younger sister.

After the Biles family relocated to Spring, Texas, Ron and Nellie gave Simone a nurturing environment that helped her grow. Simone frequently refers to Nellie as her mother. She taught her children the qualities of hard work, tenacity, and faith, all of which were crucial to Simone's path.

Learning About Gymnastics Simone's foray into gymnastics was somewhat coincidental. When she was six years old, she was enthralled by the gymnasts practicing at Bannon's Gymnastix in Houston during a field trip from her daycare. The coaches noticed Simone as she effortlessly replicated their movements. Her promise was noted by the coaches, who recommended that she take gymnastics lessons.

Mary A.Clapp

Simone started training at Bannon's Gymnastix with her family's support, and she soon showed remarkable talent and a love for the sport. Simone advanced quickly while working with coach Aimee Boorman. Early instruction placed a strong emphasis on self-control, technical proficiency, and artistic expression.

Her competition routines were eventually defined by her force and boldness, which were her well-known qualities. Simone's dedication to gymnastics intensified, and she started practicing hard. She frequently spent up to 32 hours a week at the gym while juggling homeschooling to complete her coursework.

Overcoming Obstacles Although Simone had obvious aptitude, there were challenges in her path. She had financial difficulties as a young gymnast, which frequently prevented her from attending elite training centres and competitions. But her family's constant love and sacrifice made sure she had the means to follow her aspirations.

As her skill was more widely acknowledged, Simone also had to deal with the pressure to live up to expectations and learn how to handle the psychological and emotional difficulties that come with competing in sports. Making the decision to devote herself entirely to gymnastics was one of the major turning points in her early career. Her desire to be successful on the international scene grew along with her effort.

Simone's desire to win an Olympic medal was stoked by watching gymnasts like Nastia Liukin and Shawn Johnson compete in the 2008 Beijing Olympics.

 Making the Choice to Take Gymnastics Seriously As Simone went from recreational training to competitive competition, her dedication to gymnastics was clear.

Simone started competing nationally at the age of 14, taking part in competitions like the American Classic and the U.S. Traditional. She was distinguished from her colleagues by the extraordinary difficulty and artistry of her performances. Simone first gained national attention when she participated in the Visa Championships in 2011. Her talent was evident even though she placed third in the junior division's all-around competition.

Her ambition to compete at the highest levels in gymnastics was cemented by this experience. Simone

Mary A.Clapp

relocated to the World Champions Centre, a family-owned gym in Spring, Texas, after realising she needed specialised training. There, she could hone her skills and train in cutting-edge facilities.

She created distinctive routines with the help of her trainers that highlighted her talents, especially her strong tumbling passes and creative combinations. The background and early years of Simone Biles prepared the audience for her incredible gymnastics adventure.

 Overcoming obstacles in her personal and financial life, she showed incredible talent and unwavering commitment to her sport. Simone set off on a journey that would make her one of the most renowned gymnasts in history, helped along by her family and coaches. Her early life challenges helped to form the resilient and driven athlete she is today and set the stage for her extraordinary career.

EARLY LIFE IN COLUMBUS,

Mary A.Clapp

 Ohio, was crucial in moulding Simone Biles into the tenacious and resilient person she is today. Simone was born on March 14, 1997, and lived her early years in this Midwestern city, embracing the joys and trials that would eventually shape her destiny in gymnastics and other endeavors.

 Early Struggles and Family Dynamics Simone was born into a family that was going through a lot of struggles. Because of her mother's addiction, there was instability in the family. Consequently, at the age of three, Simone and her siblings, Ashley, Tevin, and Adria, were placed in foster care.

While there was a lot of uncertainty and upheaval at this time, Simone's flexibility and fortitude were also established. Simone was raised in a close-knit family that emphasised love and support despite these early hardships. Ron Biles, her maternal grandfather, and his spouse, Nellie, were essential in offering security and nurturing. They took the enormously important step of adopting Simone and her younger sister Adria in 2000, providing them with a loving home that placed a strong emphasis on learning, self-control, and tenacity.

Relocating to Spring, Texas When Simone was six years old in 2003, the Biles family relocated to Spring, Texas, from Columbus, Ohio. Simone and her siblings were given new beginnings and chances as a result of their relocation. Simone's growing gymnastics career would take place against the backdrop of Spring, which is close to Houston. Moving to Texas also required adjusting to a new social and cultural environment.

Simone, though, rapidly adjusted to her new environment, making friends and locating a group of people who encouraged her to pursue her athletic goals. Her proximity to top-notch gymnastics training facilities and coaches who could identify and develop her potential made the relocation advantageous.

Learning and Private Schooling During her early school years, Simone attended public schools and balanced her studies with her developing interest in gymnastics. Simone and her family decided to move to homeschooling when her training needs grew, since it gave her the flexibility she needed to concentrate on her sport.

Mary A.Clapp

Simone was able to keep up a strict training regimen because of homeschooling; she frequently spent up to 32 hours a week at the gym. Simone thrived academically despite the strenuous programme, showing the same commitment to her schoolwork as she showed to gymnastics. Her capacity to strike a balance in both spheres of her life demonstrated her strong work ethic and driven ambition.

Learning About Gymnastics It was by coincidence that Simone was introduced to gymnastics. Simone was enthralled with the gymnasts she saw at Bannon's Gymnastix in Houston when she was on a field trip for childcare. She attracted the attention of the gym's teachers by effortlessly copying their moves after becoming intrigued.

The coaches were impressed by her innate talent and recommended that she take classes, which started her on a journey that would result in remarkable achievements. Simone commenced her training at Bannon's Gymnastix with her family's support. Her coaches saw her extraordinary potential right away, praising her power, agility, and fearlessness.

Early gymnastics experiences for Simone were full of victories and struggles as she learned to deal with the demands of the sport and laid the groundwork for her success in the future.

 The Function of Family Assistance Over the course of her early years, Simone's family was crucial to her growth as a person and an athlete. Unwavering in their support, Ron and Nellie Biles frequently made sacrifices to make sure Simone had the tools and chances she needed to succeed.

Simone's life and career were guided by the ideals of hard work, tenacity, and humility that were taught to her by them. Among all of them, Nellie was a regular source of advice and support. She had been a nurse before, so she knew the value of self-control and fortitude. She taught Simone to face obstacles head-on and to have a positive outlook.

 Because of the close relationship she had with her family, Simone had a solid support network that gave her the confidence to go after her aspirations.

 Social and Cultural Factors Simone was exposed to a variety of groups and cultural influences during her upbringing in Columbus, Ohio, and her relocation to Texas. Her perspective was broadened by this diversity, which also made it easier for her to deal with the complexity of the outside world as well as the gym.

 Simone's experiences in these groups influenced her moral compass and helped her appreciate the significance of inclusivity and representation in athletics. In Columbus, Ohio, Simone Biles was raised with love, resiliency, and her family's steadfast support. Simone's trip from Ohio to Texas, despite initial obstacles, laid the groundwork for her incredible gymnastics career.

Her upbringing gave her the morals and perseverance that would eventually help her become a legend in the sport. As we go deeper into Simone's narrative, we witness how her upbringing paved the way for both her remarkable accomplishments and the enduring influence she has had on gymnastics and beyond.

THE IMPACT OF FAMILY ON HER JOURNEY

Family support and advice played a crucial role in Simone Biles' development into one of the best gymnasts of all time. From conquering early obstacles to managing the demands of top competition, Simone's family has been a crucial part of her journey, guaranteeing her success both within and outside of the gym.

 A Firm Basis The tale of Simone's family is one of tenacity and affection. She and her siblings were raised in a difficult household and had great hardships as a result of their biological mother's addiction. When Simone was just three years old, their early family life became unstable, and they ended up in foster care.

It was during this trying time that the value of family support was highlighted. Simone's maternal grandparents, Ron and Nellie Biles, intervened to offer a stable and nurturing environment after realising Simone needed it. They formally adopted Simone and Adria, her younger sister, in 2000. This choice changed the girls' lives by providing a nurturing, orderly, and supportive environment.

Future achievement for Simone was made possible by Ron and Nellie's dedication to giving her a good upbringing. The Biles family made a significant relocation from Columbus, Ohio, to Spring, Texas, in 2003. Due to her migration, Simone was able to practice with top-notch gymnastics coaches and facilities, which was essential to her full potential development.

It also offered a fresh start in a new setting, where Simone's budding potential could be fully developed by the family. Throughout this change, Ron and Nellie Biles played a crucial role in making sure Simone had every chance to succeed. They understood how critical it was to encourage her gymnastics endeavours while also taking a balanced approach to her education and personal growth.

Guidance and Values from Parents Simone's adoptive mother, Nellie Biles, was especially important in establishing principles that have been crucial to Simone's personality. Nellie, a former nurse and

Mary A.Clapp

businesswoman, highlighted the value of self-control, diligence, and morality.

She encouraged Simone to stay grounded despite her rising celebrity status and taught her the importance of resilience in the face of adversity. Nellie raised Simone with an emphasis on independence and resiliency, in addition to encouraging her to succeed.

Simone has carried the principles of humility and thankfulness with her throughout her career, which she and Ron instilled in her.

 The Strength of Giving Up Simone's accomplishments in gymnastics are also evidence of the hardships her family endured. Ron and Nellie saw her extraordinary talent and committed time, effort, and money to her training. To meet Simone's rigorous training regimen, they frequently took on multiple jobs and adjusted their schedules, making sure she had the resources she needed to follow her aspirations.

The family's commitment to Simone's gymnastics career is further demonstrated by their choice to establish the cutting-edge training facility

Mary A.Clapp

World Champions Centre in Spring, Texas. In addition to offering Simone a top-notch training setting, this facility allowed other young athletes to follow their dreams of becoming gymnasts.

 Moral and Emotional Assistance In addition to providing Simone with material and financial support, her family has consistently provided emotional and ethical support. They have supported her through victories and disappointments, providing help and direction when required.

Simone has needed this constant support to help her deal with the demands of public attention and elite competition. Simone's family supported her during difficult moments, such as when she made the decision to put her mental health above her physical performance in the Tokyo 2020 Olympics, and they emphasised the value of looking after oneself in addition to one's physical accomplishments.

Their comprehension and compassion have been important throughout Simone's journey, enabling her to develop not only as an athlete but also as a person.

Her Sister Adria and Her Bond The bond that Simone has with Adria, her younger sister, has also been very important in her life. Adria, who also followed gymnastics, is very close to Simone and offers support and insight into the particular challenges experienced by professional athletes. As they encourage and support one another in their individual pursuits, their sisterly relationship has served as a source of solace and inspiration.

Influence of Extended Families Important individuals in Simone's life have also included her extended family, which consists of her biological siblings and other relatives. Her sense of self and belonging has been bolstered by the love and support of her entire family.

They have encouraged her and praised her accomplishments, highlighting the significance of family relationships in her life. It is impossible to overestimate how much Simone Biles' family influenced her life. Simone has been given the necessary foundation by Ron and Nellie Biles through their love, sacrifices, and support, which has allowed her to flourish in gymnastics and pave the way for future generations. Simone has been guided throughout her journey by their emphasis on morals, hard work, and resilience, which has enabled her to overcome obstacles and achieve incredible achievement. As we learn more about Simone's life, it becomes evident that her family's influence played a major role in both her extraordinary accomplishments and her long-lasting influence on the gymnastics community and beyond.

CHAPTER 2: DISCOVERING GYMNASTICS

Gymnast Simone Biles's path into the sport was both accidental and life-changing, launching her into an incredible career. Her early exposure to the sport laid the groundwork for her eventual ascent to the status of a gymnastics icon.

The Field Trip That Revolutionised My Life At six years old, Simone Biles went on a field trip with her daycare to Bannon's Gymnastix in Houston, Texas, where she was first introduced to gymnastics. Her life's course would abruptly alter as a result of the visit. Simone watched the athletes flip and tumble around the gym, mesmerised, while the other kids played.

 Simone couldn't resist the sport's attraction and started copying the gymnasts' enthusiastic and naturally agile routines. The coaches at the gym noticed her surprise talent exhibition and saw her potential right away. They recommended that she take gymnastics classes, which would be the catalyst for Simone's lifelong love of the sport.

 Your First Moves in the Gym Simone's parents signed her up for gymnastics lessons at Bannon's Gymnastix, per the trainers' advice. It was evident right away that Simone had a remarkable innate talent for gymnastics. She stood out from her colleagues with her strength, agility, and fearlessness, demonstrating her unique talent.

Simone started her official training in the sport with Aimee Boorman as her first instructor. Boorman saw Simone's promise right away and set out to help her grow both as a skill and as a person. Early training entailed learning the fundamentals of gymnastics and progressively working up to increasingly difficult routines that would highlight Simone's special abilities.

 Early Difficulties and Triumphs Although Simone's talent was immediately apparent, she had a number of difficulties in her early training. Financial limitations were a major obstacle because gymnastics instruction can be costly and involves paying for coaching, gear, and competition costs. Despite these obstacles, Simone's family was willing to make compromises in order to help her develop professionally, since they knew how important it was to fulfil her potential. Simone also had to figure out how to reconcile her academic pursuits with the physical demands of gymnastics.

She went to public school at first, but as her training got more intense, her family realised that homeschooling would give her the flexibility she needed to meet her demanding training schedule. Despite these difficulties, Simone experienced many breakthroughs and self-discovering moments during her early gymnastics years. Her love of the game strengthened her resolve, and she advanced through the ranks fast, winning praise for her outstanding achievements in regional tournaments.

 Locating a Guide Simone's first gymnast coach, Aimee Boorman, was a major influence in her early training. Boorman worked hard to develop Simone's passion for the game, in addition to helping her improve her abilities. She created a loving and encouraging atmosphere that let Simone grow and discover her potential fearlessly. Simone started to refine her trademark style—a blend of strong athleticism and avant-garde artistry—under Boorman's tutelage.

Boorman laid the foundation for Simone's future success by encouraging her to play to her strengths and push the limits of what was thought to be achievable in gymnastics. Ascending the hierarchy, Simone started competing in regional and national events, which was a sign that her commitment and diligence were paying off.

Her unusual blend of strength, accuracy, and personality made her performances regularly impressive to both judges and fans. When Simone competed at the American Classic in Houston in 2011, it was one of her first notable successes. Simone, who is relatively new to competitive gymnastics, qualified for the national finals with an impressive performance. Her rise in the gymnastics world began with her victory in this competition.

Enhancing Her Capabilities As Simone's training progressed, she concentrated on honing her abilities on the vault, uneven bars, balancing beam, and floor exercises. She distinguished herself from her contemporaries with her strong tumbling passes and creative routines, which made her a rising star in the sport. Simone's unwavering pursuit of perfection demonstrated her passion for honing her craft. She put in endless hours honing her technique and challenging herself to learn ever-more-difficult talents at the gym. Her enthusiasm for gymnastics and her dedication to training were important contributors to her quick development and success.

The Function of Family Assistance Simone's family was and has always been her biggest source of support. Her siblings and parents, Ron and Nellie Biles, were her constant supporters, providing inspiration and support. They cheered her on, supported her through difficult times, and attended her competitions. Simone was able to concentrate on her gymnastics profession with confidence and drive because of the Biles family's consistent support.

Simone's dreams were made possible by their unwavering faith in her abilities and their readiness to make concessions. When Simone Biles discovered gymnastics, it was the start of an amazing adventure filled with skill, diligence, and willpower. She was first exposed to the sport on a daycare field trip, which proved to be a turning point in her career.

Simone became an extremely strong athlete, laying the groundwork for her future as a gymnastics legend with the help of her coaches and family. As we delve deeper into Simone's narrative, we witness how her early struggles and hardships moulded her into the incredible gymnast and role model that she is today.

ENTRY POINT OF THE GYM

Mary A.Clapp

When Simone Biles initially entered the gymnastics world, she was full of enthusiasm, natural talent, and hunger to learn. She was destined for greatness from the minute she stepped foot in a gymnastics gym. Her early involvement in the sport served as a springboard for her eventual rise to become one of the greatest gymnasts of all time.

Bannon's Gymnastix: A Fresh Start Simone Biles started her official gymnastics training at Bannon's Gymnastix in Houston, Texas, following her accidental discovery of the sport while on a field trip with her daycare. From the beginning, Simone saw the gym as a second home, a place where she could explore her innate skills and fully immerse herself in the world of gymnastics. With its reputation for providing a caring atmosphere and fostering the growth of youthful talent, Bannon's Gymnastix was the ideal starting point for Simone. Simone was able to gain confidence in her skills and learn the principles of gymnastics in a friendly environment at the club.

Aimee Boorman, Coach: A Directing Force Simone was matched with Aimee Boorman at Bannon's Gymnastix, who would go on to play a significant role in both her personal and professional life. Boorman noticed in Simone a special blend of athleticism, charisma, and dedication, and he spotted her remarkable potential right away. Aimee Boorman's coaching method placed equal emphasis on cultivating a love of the sport and forging a close bond between the athlete and the coach, in addition to honing technical skills.

She was aware of how critical it was to establish a supportive and upbeat atmosphere so Simone could flourish. Simone started learning the foundations of gymnastics from Boorman. This involved becoming proficient on all of the equipment, including the floor exercise, uneven bars, vault, and balance beam. Simone's desire to learn and her commitment to honing her talents demonstrated her passion for the sport.

Early Difficulties and Willpower In spite of her innate ability, Simone had various obstacles in her early gym career. Simone had to put in a lot of effort to acquire the extreme physical strength, flexibility, and discipline needed for gymnastics. Her extraordinary power and boldness, which distinguished her from her colleagues and ultimately defined her unique style, were noted by her coaches.

During her early training, Simone focused on developing her technical skills, strength, and endurance. She spent a lot of time in the gym honing her skills, practicing routines that required focus and control. Even at a young age, her drive to persevere and her will to succeed were clear to see.

Discovering Her Individual Style As Simone's training developed, it became evident that she had a distinct style that distinguished her from other gymnasts. She attracted audiences with her unwavering personality, high-flying aerial manoeuvres, and strong tumbling passes in her routines. Early performances by Simone demonstrated her ability to combine creativity and athleticism, a combination that would later come to define her career.

Coaches and judges alike praised her for her strength and agility, especially in her spectacular floor performances. Simone was encouraged by Aimee Boorman to embrace her uniqueness and create routines that emphasised her talents. Simone was able to explore new avenues in the sport and gain confidence in her abilities thanks to this method.

The Value of Support from Family Simone's family was there for her no matter what during her early gymnastics years. Ron and Nellie Biles, her parents, saw her talent and gave up everything to make sure she had the means to follow her desire. This involved paying for her training, making plans for getting to and from the gym, and travelling to tournaments to support her.

Simone's siblings contributed significantly to her trip as well. Simone felt very much a part of the family and was inspired to keep working hard by their support and mutual excitement for her achievements. Simone's success can be attributed in large part to the Biles family's dedication to her gymnastics profession, which gave her the confidence and drive to concentrate on her training.

Quick Ascent Through the Levels Simone rose quickly in the gymnastics ranks because of her talent and diligence. She became known as a rising star in the gymnastics world as a result of her impressive results in local and regional competitions. One of Simone's first noteworthy accomplishments was participating in the American Classic in Houston in 2011.

She was very new to competitive gymnastics, but she made a great impression and qualified for the national finals. Her climb in the gymnastics world began with this accomplishment. When Simone Biles stepped foot in the Bannon's Gymnastix facility, it signalled the start of an incredible journey filled with skill, diligence, and willpower. Her early involvement in the sport served as a springboard for her eventual rise to prominence as one of the greatest gymnasts in history.

Simone took advantage of the opportunities and difficulties that came her way, paving the way for her future success and influence in gymnastics with the help of her coach and family. As we learn more about Simone's life, we can see how her early encounters and distinctive style helped to mould her into the exceptional athlete she is today.

PRIMARY COACHES AND IMPACTORS

Simone Biles's trainers and mentors, who saw her extraordinary talent and encouraged her potential, had a big influence on her early gymnastic growth. These early influences played a critical role in helping Simone hone her abilities, create her distinct style, and lay the groundwork for her career as a top gymnast.

Aimee Boorman: Encouraging Spirit One of the most important people in Simone Biles' early gymnastics career was Aimee Boorman, who served as her first coach. When Simone joined Bannon's Gymnastix in Houston, Texas, at the age of six, that's when their connection started. Boorman observed Simone's inherent potential right away and saw in her a unique blend of charisma, athleticism, and determination.

Coaching Theory: Boorman's coaching method emphasised perseverance, discipline, and hard work while fostering Simone's love for the game. She was a firm believer in fostering an environment that was encouraging and helpful so that Simone could discover her potential and establish her own style. Simone was pushed to execute performances that highlighted her strength and ingenuity by Boorman, who urged her to embrace her individuality.

Creating a Robust Athlete-Coach Bond: Boorman and Simone had a close relationship that was marked by mutual respect and trust. Boorman made sure Simone felt strong and self-assured both inside and outside of the gym by striking a balance between technical instruction and emotional support. Simone and Boorman had a collaboration as he helped her through the ups and downs of her early gymnastics adventure.

New Approaches to Training: Simone's abilities on the vault, uneven bars, balancing beam, and floor exercise were greatly enhanced by Boorman. She developed cutting-edge training methods that emphasised Simone's advantages, especially her strong tumbling and daring attitude towards difficult routines. Simone was able to create technically challenging but also visually captivating routines thanks to Boorman's emphasis on emotion and originality.

Chris Burdette and Support Coaches' Role Although Simone's main coach was Aimee Boorman, several other coaches were equally important to her early growth. Chris Burdette was one such coach who co-owned Bannon's Gymnastics with Boorman. Burdette helped Simone with her training, especially with the uneven bars, which were a difficult apparatus for her at first.

Pay Attention to Technical Accuracy: Burdette helped Simone hone her abilities and develop consistency in her routines by concentrating on technical accuracy and execution. Boorman's inventive approach was enhanced by his focus on technique and attention to detail, giving Simone a well-rounded training programme that catered to every facet of her gymnastics growth.

Gymnastics Role Models' Influence Throughout her early career, Simone Biles looked up to other gymnasts who functioned as role models in addition to her coaches. The world-class gymnasts [Nastia Liukin, Shawn Johnson, and Gabby Douglas] inspired Simone to strive for perfection and her desire to compete internationally.

Shane Johnson and Natasha Liukin: For Simone, it was a turning point to watch Shawn Johnson and Nastia Liukin perform in the 2008 Beijing Olympics. She was motivated to set high standards for herself and to represent the United States in the Olympic Games by their performances. Simone used their accomplishments and commitment as a standard for her own goals.

Gabby Douglas: Simone was also greatly influenced by Gabby Douglas, the first African American gymnast to win the 2012 Olympic all-around title. Simone experienced a sense of empowerment and representation from Gabby's achievement. Simone was motivated to break down boundaries and strive for excellence because she saw in Gabby a reflection of her own potential.

Creating a Signature Look Early mentors of Simone Biles pushed her to hone a distinct technique that fused artistry, power, and precision. Simone's remarkable ability to execute challenging abilities with ease was acknowledged by Boorman and her crew, who encouraged her to add creative elements to her routines.

Strength and Agility: Strong tumbling passes and daring aerial movements made Simone's routines famous. She stood out from her colleagues thanks to her outstanding height and amplitude of skills, which were made possible by her athleticism. Coaches stressed the importance of using this strength to produce technically challenging and striking routines.

Creative Expression: Simone's trainers urged her to express herself artistically in her performances, in addition to her athletic skill. Simone was able to connect with judges and viewers by putting her artistic focus first, which gave her routines a deeper emotional quality. Her signature style was her ability to blend grace and strength, which made her one of gymnastics' most compelling performers.

Overcoming Obstacles Simone had numerous difficulties in her early gymnastics years, despite her talent. Two major obstacles were the sport's physical demands and financial limitations. She overcame these challenges, though, with the help and direction of her instructors, who gave her the perseverance and tenacity she needed to be successful.

Money Difficulties: Training in gymnastics is costly since it involves fees for tournaments, coaching, and equipment. Simone's trainers were crucial in figuring out how to give her the chances she required to succeed, even if her family had to make sacrifices to support her career.

Mental and Physical Demands: Gymnastics has extremely high physical requirements, involving strength, flexibility, and endurance. Simone's coaches helped her develop the physical toughness required for the sport by emphasising the value of fitness and preventing injuries. They also offered Simone emotional support, which helped her build the mental toughness required to withstand the demands of elite sports.

Early mentors and influencers had a significant impact on Simone Biles's gymnastic career. Aimee Boorman and other encouraging coaches helped Simone grow into a formidable athlete whose distinct style enthralled spectators all over the world.

Her will to succeed was fueled by the support and motivation she received from her coaches as well as the role models she looked up to, which paved the way for her future successes. As we delve deeper into Simone's story, it becomes clearer how these early inspirations shaped her extraordinary career and her long-lasting influence on the gymnastics community.

CHAPTER 3: OVERCOMING CHALLENGES

There were many obstacles in Simone Biles' path to gymnastics fame, both personal and professional. She has a solid support network around her, resilience, and tenacity, all of which have contributed to her capacity to overcome these challenges. From early misfortune to the demands of top competition, Simone overcame a range of challenges that moulded her path and cemented her reputation as a gymnastics icon.

Family Difficulties Early in life, Simone Biles faced numerous difficulties as a result of her familial circumstances. Due to her original mother's addiction, Simone and her siblings were put into foster care. Her life drastically changed when she was taken in by Ron and Nellie Biles, her grandparents, and placed in foster care. The Biles family gave Simone a caring and encouraging environment that was essential for her development, despite the unpredictability.

Budgetary Restrictions Significant financial resources were needed for Simone's ascent in gymnastics. Due to the high expenses of competition, coaching, and training, her family had difficulty affording to support her developing career. Ron and Nellie Biles gave up a lot to make sure Simone could follow her dream, and they frequently went above and beyond to help her prepare for contests.

GYMNASTICS' PHYSICAL DEMANDS

Physical strains and injuries Because gymnastics requires such high physical standards, Simone Biles had numerous physical setbacks and injuries during her career. Simone experienced problems early in her career, including injuries to her ankles and wrists that needed medical care and rehabilitation.

Mary A.Clapp

The sport's extreme physical demands required meticulous injury management in addition to a demanding training schedule. Simone's ability to bounce back from these injuries and compete at a higher level demonstrated her tenacity. Her commitment to injury avoidance, training, and close collaboration with medical specialists was essential to handling the physical demands of the sport.

 Juggling Education and Training Simone found it more and more difficult to balance her demanding training routine with her schooling as her gymnastics career developed. After attending public school for a while, Simone's family opted to homeschool her in order to meet her rigorous training schedule.

Simone was able to continue her academic obligations and devote more time to gymnastics as a result of this decision. The obstacles of homeschooling were unique in that Simone needed to learn time management skills to succeed in the classroom and the gym. Her capacity to manage these obligations revealed her strong work ethic and dedication to her objectives.

ELITE COMPETITION'S PRESSURES

Emotional and Mental Stress Gymnasts that compete at the top levels go through a lot of mental and emotional strain. Simone Biles was under constant media, fan, and rival criticism. She had extra pressure to perform well because of the expectations put on her, especially since she was the favourite to win the Olympic gold medal. Simone's success depended heavily on her capacity to handle this pressure. She worked with sports psychologists to preserve mental toughness and focus, among other coping mechanisms, to manage the psychological pressures of competition.

The 2020 Tokyo Olympics One of Simone's biggest obstacles came during the Olympics in Tokyo 2020, when she bravely chose to put her mental well-being ahead of her performance. Following a bout of "twisties," a disorder impacting her coordination and spatial awareness, Simone made the decision to miss a few events in order to protect her health and safety. Both praise and criticism were directed towards this choice. The significance of mental health in athletics was brought to light by Simone's courageous decision to openly discuss her mental health issues. Her choice to back off showed maturity and self-awareness and also advanced the discussion on athletes' mental health in general.

The Family's Function Despite all of her difficulties, Simone's family was there for her always. Simone received financial, logistical, and emotional support from Ron and Nellie Biles as they helped her through the highs and lows of her gymnastics career. She was able to overcome challenges and concentrate on her objectives because of their support and sacrifices. Simone's family's close-knit support system enabled her to stay motivated and stable, which in turn gave her the confidence and fortitude to overcome obstacles.

Guidance Assistance Aimee Boorman and other coaches were instrumental in assisting Simone in overcoming obstacles. They assisted Simone in managing the demands of elite competition and helping her deal with physical injuries by offering direction, encouragement, and technical support. Her capacity to endure despite challenges was greatly influenced by their devotion to her development and conviction in her potential. Simone Biles faced several difficulties along the way that put her fortitude, tenacity, and strength to the test before she became a gymnastics icon.

Simone confronted every challenge head-on, from overcoming early personal setbacks to handling the mental and physical strain of elite competition. She did it with bravery and determination. She overcame these obstacles and accomplished remarkable achievements with the help of her family, coaches, and her own inner drive. As we go deeper into Simone's narrative, we observe how her perseverance has been a distinguishing characteristic of her extraordinary career and enduring influence on the gymnastics community.

Personal Difficulties and Achievements In addition to her amazing accomplishments, Simone Biles' path to becoming a gymnastics superstar is characterised by the challenges she overcame personally. Her tale is one of tenacity, bravery, and success, showing how she overcame obstacles inside and outside of the gym to reach success.

Foster care and family instability: Because of the difficulties her biological mother faced with addiction, Simone had a difficult childhood. Simone and her siblings were placed in foster care as a result of this turmoil. Simone's final adoption by her grandparents, Ron and Nellie Biles, gave her a secure and nurturing environment that was essential for her growth, despite the challenges of being in foster care.

Budgetary Restrictions Pursuing a gymnastics career came with substantial financial costs. The expenses of Simone's competition, coaching, and training were a burden on her family. In order to finance Simone's gymnastics career, Ron and Nellie Biles had to make significant sacrifices. They frequently worked multiple jobs and closely monitored their finances to make sure Simone had the training supplies she required.

Overcoming Obstacles of the Body Due to the strenuous physical requirements of gymnastics, Simone sustained multiple injuries over her career. Her wrists and ankles suffered early injuries that necessitated medical care and rehabilitation. Simone's fortitude was put to the test each time she sustained an injury, necessitating periods of rest and recuperation before she could resume her best work. Simone's physical toughness and tenacity were demonstrated by her ability to bounce back from setbacks and carry on with her excellent performance. Her dedication to injury avoidance and conditioning helped her cope with the demanding physical demands of the sport.

Tokyo 2020's "Twisties" The Olympics in Tokyo 2020 posed one of Simone's biggest obstacles. Simone contracted the "twisties," a disorder that impairs an athlete's coordination and spatial awareness, during the Games. She could not safely do complicated gymnastics routines because of this problem. Simone made the tough choice to miss a few events in order to put her physical and mental health first. Her openness about her battle with the twisties emphasised her bravery in tackling such challenges and raised awareness of the significance of mental health in athletics.

Psychological and Emotional Difficulties As a prominent gymnastics personality, Simone was subject to intense scrutiny and high standards from the general public, the media, and herself. Being a top athlete came with a lot of demands and scrutiny, which frequently caused severe emotional stress. It took strong mental fortitude and the capacity to stay focused in the face of outside challenges to handle this pressure. In order to retain her mental resilience, Simone developed coping mechanisms and collaborated with sports psychologists to manage this stress. Her psychological fortitude was evident in her capacity to perform well under duress and maintain concentration during tournaments.

Juggling Notoriety with Personal Life Being famous at an early age came with its own set of difficulties. Simone had to balance her desire for seclusion and normalcy with navigating the intricacies of public life. Her family and team had to provide her with careful guidance and support as she juggled the demands of her gymnastics career with her personal life. Simone used firm boundaries and a grounded approach to control her public persona. Her close friends and family were extremely important in assisting her in balancing the demands of celebrity with her commitment to gymnastics and her own health.

VICTORIES AND ACCOMPLISHMENTS

Gymnastics Breakthroughs Simone has had a number of noteworthy victories over her career. Her early triumphs in local, state, and national contests prepared the ground for her subsequent successes. Her maiden major triumph came in the 2013 World Championships, starting a run of wins that included multiple World Championships and Olympic gold. Her achievements at the 2016 Rio Olympics, when she took home four golds and one bronze, cemented her reputation as a gymnastics icon. As one of the best gymnasts of all time, Simone gained international recognition for her ability to execute inventive routines with remarkable precision and artistry.

Effect on Athletics and Other Domains Beyond just her sporting prowess, Simone has a significant influence. For young athletes, especially those from marginalised backgrounds, she has emerged as a role model. She has become a strong advocate for reform and advancement in the gymnastics community due to her candour about her battles with mental health and her support of changes in the sport. In addition to her incredible feats, Simone has made a lasting impact on gymnastics through her efforts to encourage and assist other athletes.

Her legacy includes promoting a more open and friendly atmosphere for athletes as well as a better knowledge of mental health issues. The narrative of Simone Biles as a gymnastics legend is inextricably linked to her personal difficulties and victories. Simone has shown incredible bravery and fortitude, handling both physical disabilities and emotional difficulties in addition to overcoming early family hardships and financial limitations.

Her accomplishments on the international scene are evidence of her perseverance, hard work, and capacity to overcome hardship. When we consider Simone's trajectory, we see a wonderful athlete who has not only excelled in gymnastics but also used her platform to inspire people all around the world and have a lasting impact on the sport.

THE CHOICE TO TAKE A SERIOUS LOOK AT GYMNASTICS

A turning point in Simone Biles' life was when she decided to take gymnastics seriously. It turned her from a young, talented gymnast to an elite athlete with immense potential. Her innate talent, her family's backing, and her personal enthusiasm for the sport all played a part in this decision.

NATURAL TALENT AND EARLY PASSION

The Gymnastics Discovery Simone developed a strong interest in gymnastics after her first experience with the sport on a field trip to Bannon's Gymnastix for her daycare. Her potential was evident from her first fascination and natural ability to mimic gymnastic moves. Her parents enrolled her in gymnastics classes after seeing her early talent, which laid the groundwork for her eventual serious dedication to the discipline.

Motivation from Coaches Simone's extraordinary abilities were instantly recognised by her coaches at Bannon's Gymnastix. Simone's first instructor, Aimee Boorman, was instrumental in igniting her passion and commitment to gymnastics. Simone's decision to take gymnastics seriously was greatly influenced by Boorman's support and faith in her abilities.

FAMILY ASSISTANCE AND GIVING

Ron and Nellie Biles's Roles Simone's decision to concentrate on gymnastics was greatly influenced by her grandparents, Ron and Nellie Biles. Their steadfast assistance involved them making large monetary and non-material sacrifices in order to provide Simone with the tools and chances she needed to succeed in the sport. Simone's decision to take gymnastics seriously was greatly influenced by their dedication to her training and health.

Juggling Gymnastics and Family The Biles family was more than willing to make material sacrifices. They gave Simone emotional support and stability so she could concentrate on her training without having to worry about her family's instability. Simone made the decision to devote herself entirely to gymnastics because of her solid familial support network.

THE SHIFT TO ELITE INSTRUCTION

Transitioning to National Contests Simone started competing in gymnastics competitions at the regional and national levels as her abilities and performances increased. Her determination to take gymnastics seriously was strengthened by her success in these contests, which included standout performances at the American Classic. Simone's motivation to keep improving in the sport came from each victory and accolade. The choice to homeschool: Simone and her family chose to go from public to homeschooling in order to meet her rigorous training schedule. The need for more flexibility and time to devote to gymnastics led to this decision. Simone's homeschooling helped her to manage both her demanding training schedule and her academic obligations, which strengthened her dedication to the sport.

MOTIVATORS AND INFLUENCES

Gymnastics Role Models Famous gymnasts like Gabby Douglas, Shawn Johnson, and Nastia Liukin served as inspiration for Simone. Simone was inspired by their Olympic accomplishments and success to pursue her own goals of competing internationally. Seeing these role models reach greatness gave Simone a clear idea of what was attainable and strengthened her will to be successful.

Ambitions and Personal Goals Simone decided to take gymnastics seriously since it fit with her personal aims and aspirations. She gave her all to her training since she loved the sport and wanted to compete at the top levels. Simone chose to concentrate on gymnastics because she was driven by her desire to succeed and leave her mark in the sport.

GETTING PAST CHALLENGES

Overcoming Setbacks There were challenges along the way to becoming an outstanding gymnast. Simone had to deal with a number of difficulties, such as limited resources, bodily harm, and competitive pressures. Her determination to pursue gymnastics in spite of these difficulties demonstrated her tenacity and commitment.

Seizing the Chances Simone's decision to study gymnastics seriously was greatly influenced by her capacity to identify and seize possibilities for personal growth and development. She used competitive chances, coaching, and training to further her career and improve her talents. One of the turning points in Simone Biles' life was her choice to do gymnastics seriously.

Mary A.Clapp

With the help of her family, personal aspirations, and innate talent, Simone developed from a young, talented gymnast into a top athlete with a clear understanding of her objectives. Her passion and dedication to gymnastics are demonstrated by her perseverance in the face of adversity. Looking at Simone's trajectory, we can see how this crucial choice paved the way for her incredible accomplishments and enduring influence on the sport.

CHAPTER 4: RISE TO STARDOM-JUNIOR COMPETITION YEARS

During her junior competitive years, Simone Biles turned heads with her outstanding results. She was developing as a gymnast, and this was the time to show off her incredible potential and set the foundation for her future success.

 Premiere at the 2011 American Classic In the competitive gymnastics world, Simone Biles made her debut at the 2011 American Classic in Houston, Texas. She was relatively new on the national scene, but her performance was exceptional and showed her promise. She qualified for the national championships and received attention for her performance at this competition.

First-ever National Achievement Simone participated in the U.S. National Championships in 2011 and gained notoriety for her impressive results there. She showed that she could perform well under duress and carry out intricate routines with accuracy. Her rise in the gymnastics world began with her impressive performance at the national championships.

Groundbreaking Acts 2012 Junior National Championships in the U.S. For Simone, the 2012 U.S. Junior National Championships marked a sea change in her career. She became a formidable force, taking home gold in the vault and floor exercise as well as the all-around championship. Her success in this competition cemented her as an emerging gymnastics star.

Global Premiere Simone competed in the 2012 Pacific Rim Championships in Seattle, demonstrating her excellence in junior tournaments. She demonstrated her abilities there by taking home several medals, including gold in the vault, floor exercise, and all-around competitions. Her readiness to compete at the highest levels was proved by her international success, which also established her as a gymnast to watch.

SIGNATURE SKILL DEVELOPMENT

Specializing in Difficult Tasks Simone's distinctive routines, which are marked by precise skills and high-flying tumbling passes, were developed and honed during her junior years. Her performances stood out from the rest of her contemporaries due to their difficulty and execution. Simone's signature style was her ability to execute difficult and inventive sequences with strength and grace.

Pay Attention to Specific Events Due to her early training and competitive experience, Simone was able to concentrate on honing her abilities on the vault, uneven bars, balancing beam, and floor exercises. She achieved significant progress in every category, but especially in the floor and vault exercises, where she started using characteristic movements that would eventually become her signatures.

OVERCOMING DIFFICULTIES AT THE JUNIOR LEVEL

Juggling Personal Life and Training The journey from a young competitor to an elite gymnast required juggling demanding training schedules with personal obligations. In order to manage her training schedule and make sure she had the resources and stability she needed, Simone's family's support was essential. She had to exercise a great deal of discipline and dedication at this time to meet the demands of elite competition.

Adjusting to Increased Levels of Competition Simone had to adjust to increasing levels of competition as her career progressed. Meets at the junior level were followed by national and international competitions that got harder and harder. Simone's development as a gymnast depended heavily on her capacity to rise to these new obstacles and maintain her high caliber of performance.

ACKNOWLEDGMENT AND AWARDS

Recognition on a National Scale Because of her junior year results, Simone received a lot of praise and respect from the gymnastics community. Coaches, the media, and fans took notice of her accomplishments at national events, which made her a household name among the nation's best young gymnasts.

Global Accomplishments Simone's achievements went beyond national boundaries, as she kept making an impression in international contests. Her rising stature as a competitive gymnast was aided by her triumphs at the Pacific Rim Championships and other international events. These accomplishments gave her exposure to the international arena and invaluable experience.

MAKING THE SWITCH TO SENIOR COMPETITION

Senior Level Readiness Simone started getting ready for the move as she got closer to the age at which she could compete at the senior level. This required her to modify her training so that it concentrated on the harder and more intense senior events. Simone's successful transition to senior competition was largely attributed to her unwavering commitment to honing her routines and talents.

Mary A.Clapp

 Initial Senior Contests Simone made her senior competition debut in the 2013 U.S. National Championships, where she carried on her junior year success. Her performances at these competitions showed that she was prepared to compete at the top levels and hinted at what she might do in the future. The junior competition years of Simone Biles were characterized by remarkable accomplishments, remarkable talent, and outstanding performances.

 Her achievements during this time demonstrated her ability to compete at the top levels of gymnastics, laying the groundwork for her eventual prominence. Simone's commitment, skill growth, and outstanding accomplishments during the junior-to-senior competition laid the groundwork for her subsequent ascent to notoriety in the gymnastics community.

Early Runs and Remarkable Successes Early competitive years for Simone Biles were characterized by a string of outstanding performances and noteworthy triumphs that solldified her status as a rising star in the gymnastics community. Her triumphs in these contests demonstrated her extraordinary talent and paved the way for her future achievements.

FIRST CONTESTS

American Classic (2011) At Houston, Texas's 2011 American Classic, Simone Biles left a lasting impression. Simone was up against a lot of skilled gymnasts, but judges and coaches were impressed by her achievements. Her memorable routines showed off her promise and offered a sneak peek at the extraordinary talent that would characterize her career.

(2011) U.S. National Championships Simone Biles gave a national stage performance at the 2011 U.S. National Championships. She started to be recognized for her powerful routines and potential after turning in some outstanding results in the junior class. Her first foray into elite-level gymnastics with this tournament laid the groundwork for her subsequent achievements. L

GROUNDBREAKING TRIUMPHS

Junior National Championships held in the US (2012) For Simone Biles, the 2012 U.S. Junior National

Championships marked a turning point. She won the all-around competition, showcasing her adaptability and talent on every apparatus. She also won gold medals on the floor exercise and vault, solidifying her position as the dominant force in junior gymnastics.

Championships Around the Pacific (2012) Simone's success continued in the international arena, as demonstrated in Seattle at the 2012 Pacific Rim Championships. Simone competed against athletes from around the world and won gold in the vault, floor exercise, and all-around events. Her accomplishments at this meet demonstrated how well-known she is becoming as one of the world's best young gymnasts.

ONGOING ACHIEVEMENT AND ACKNOWLEDGMENT

U.S. National Championships in 2013 Simone Biles carried on her stellar performance at the 2013 U.S. National Championships. She took home the gold in vault and floor exercise, as well as the all-around crown in the senior class, thanks to her amazing performances. Her promotion to senior-level gymnastics and continued recognition as a top gymnast were both marked by this tournament.

International Competitions (2013) Simone's triumph at the 2013 World Championships in Antwerp, Belgium, was her latest international achievement. She became the first African American gymnast to win the gold medal in the all-around competition. Simone also won bronze on the balance beam and gold medals on the vault and floor exercises. Her achievement at these championships hinted at her potential for future supremacy in the sport and showed that she could compete at the highest levels.

NOTABLE VICTORIES AND ACCOMPLISHMENTS

America's Classic 2014: Simone Biles continued to be a top gymnast at the 2014 U.S. Classic with another outstanding performance. In addition to winning the gold medals in vault, floor exercise, and balance beam, she also won the all-around title. Her performance at this meet cemented her as one of the nation's top gymnasts even further.

Mary A.Clapp

World Championships of 2014 Simone Biles kept winning at the 2014 World Championships in Nanning, China. She took home gold in the vault, balance beam, floor exercise, and all-around competitions. Her outstanding accomplishments at these championships confirmed her place among the best gymnasts in the world and paved the way for more achievements.

Initial Successes and Legacy Early contests and noteworthy victories for Simone Biles proved her extraordinary talent and laid the groundwork for her future professional endeavors. Her accomplishments in both national and international competitions demonstrated her adaptability, talent, and capacity for high-pressure performance. These early triumphs made Simone a well-known personality in gymnastics and helped to shape the path for her future success and influence in the discipline.

Early contests and significant victories for Simone Biles played a pivotal role in molding her career and solidifying her status as a gymnastics icon. Her tremendous skill was exposed, and the groundwork for her future accomplishments was laid by her outstanding performances in national and international events. When we consider Simone's early accomplishments, we can see how her initial successes and notoriety prepared the way for her incredible career in the gymnastics world.

ESTABLISHING A RECORD AS A RISING STAR

The ability to establish herself as a rising star was a key factor in Simone Biles' rise to fame in gymnastics. Her outstanding competitive results, impressive skill set, and extraordinary performances all contributed to her being recognized as one of the most promising gymnasts of her generation.

Initial Thoughts and Unique Abilities Special Passes and Routines for Tumbling Simone Biles had a distinct and strong style from the start of her competitive career. She distinguishes herself from other gymnasts with her intricate twists and high-flying talents during her tumbling passes. Coaches, competitors, and judges all praised Simone for her ability to execute these challenging sequences with grace and precision.

Gymnastics' Innovations Simone's routines were known for their inventive components and challenging talents that were seldom seen in other performances. She pushed the limits of gymnastics with new combinations and changes in her performances. These inventions demonstrated not only her inventiveness but also her ability as a gymnast to redefine the sport.

NOTABLE TOURNAMENTS AND SUCCESSES

Championships for the United States (2013-2015) The **U.S. National Championships** triumph for Simone was a major contributor to her rise to fame. Her triumphs in 2013, 2014, and 2015 proved her superiority and consistency in the field. Simone's yearly achievements cemented her position as a top contender, garnering her acclaim and honors within the gymnastics community.

Global Acknowledgment Simone's reputation was further reinforced by her performances on the world stage. Her accomplishments in the World Championships in 2013 and 2014 demonstrated her capacity to contend with and outperform the world's top gymnasts. Her stature was enhanced, and her preparedness for high-level competition was proven by her international triumphs.

PUBLIC PERCEPTION AND MEDIA EXPOSURE

News and Highlights Simone's outstanding performances and increasing popularity garnered a lot of media attention. Her popularity grew as a result of the widespread coverage of her accomplishments and memorable performances. Her accomplishments were emphasized by media sources and gymnastics aficionados, which aided in establishing her reputation as a rising star.

Public persona and role model In addition to her accomplishments, Simone has a warm and engaging personality that has helped her connect with fans and motivate aspiring gymnasts. She became a role model for future athletes due to her commitment to the sport and her upbeat public image, which further cemented her status as a budding gymnastics star.

ASSISTANCE AND GUIDANCE

Mentoring and Instruction The direction and mentorship Simone received from her coaches also contributed to her success. Her early coach, Aimee Boorman, was important in helping her hone her abilities and get ready for competition. With Boorman's guidance and encouragement, Simone was able to hone her routines and perform at her best, which enhanced her standing as a great gymnast.

Support for Families Simone's family's steadfast support was crucial to her path. Her grandparents, Ron and Nellie Biles, provide emotional support in addition to material and administrative assistance. Because of their dedication to her achievement, Simone was able to concentrate on her training and keep establishing herself as a rising star.

EFFECT ON ATHLETICS

Establishing New Parameters Gymnasts now hold higher standards because of Simone's inventiveness and performances. Her extraordinary skill and execution of intricate routines pushed other gymnasts to improve their own performances. Beyond her personal accomplishments, Simone had a significant impact on the sport, changing and improving gymnastics routines and methods.

 Motivating the Upcoming Generation Young gymnasts all throughout the world found inspiration in Simone's ascent to fame. Her accomplishments and commitment inspired young athletes to follow their own goals by showcasing the opportunities in the sport. Simone's position as a trailblazer and role model was further cemented by her influence on the upcoming generation of gymnasts.

Rising star status for Simone Biles was earned through noteworthy accomplishments, creative routines, and outstanding performances. Her reputation as one of the most promising gymnasts of her day was cemented by her accomplishments in both national and international events, media appearances, and public image. Her impact on the sport and the encouragement she received from her coaches and family cemented her status as a budding star and paved the way for her future success and influence in gymnastics.

CHAPTER 5: SENIOR DEBUT AND BREAKTHROUGH

A turning point in Simone Biles' career occurred when she moved from junior to senior competition. This was followed by a string of ground-breaking performances that cemented her reputation as a gymnastics superstar. Her outstanding talent was on display in her senior debut, which also laid the groundwork for her incredible ascent in the sport.

SENIOR PREMIERE

Mary A.Clapp

 U.S. National Championships in 2013 In August 2013, Simone Biles debuted as a senior at the 2013 U.S. National Championships. Simone, up against a group of experienced gymnasts, stunned the gymnastics community with an incredible performance. She proved her adaptability and skill on all four apparatuses—the vault, uneven bars, balance beam, and floor exercise—to win the all-around title. Simone also won gold medals in floor exercises and vault, which emphasizes even more of her extraordinary skills.

 Global Effect Simone's accomplishments at international tournaments defined her senior debut. A major turning point in her career came at the 2013 World Championships in Antwerp, Belgium. Simone became the first African American gymnast to win the gold medal in the all-around competition. Her vault, floor exercise, and balance beam efforts brought her gold medals as well as a bronze on the balancing beam. Her ability to succeed on a worldwide scale was demonstrated by her international achievements, which also paved the way for her ongoing dominance in the sport.

GROUNDBREAKING ACCOMPLISHMENTS

Mary A.Clapp

 U.S. National Championships in 2014 At the 2014 U.S. National Championships, Simone demonstrated her unwavering dominance by winning gold medals in the vault, floor exercise, and balance beam events, in addition to repeating her all-around victory. Her accomplishments at this meet strengthened her standing as one of the nation's best gymnasts. Simone's talent and preparation were evident in her ability to execute at a high level every time and in her outstanding performances.

 World Championships of 2014 For Simone, the 2014 World Championships in Nanning, China, represented yet another milestone. She took home gold in the vault, balance beam, floor exercise, and all-around competitions. Simone's accomplishments at these championships cemented her status as one of the world's best gymnasts by showcasing her unmatched talent and adaptability. Her accomplishments at the 2014 Worlds enhanced her already-growing profile and solidified her position as the leading competitor in the world of gymnastics.

SIGNIFICANCE AND ACKNOWLEDGMENT

Asserting Control Simone Biles became a dominant force in gymnastics with her breakthrough performances and senior debut. She stands out from other gymnasts with her ability to execute intricate routines with remarkable accuracy. Simone's accomplishments in national and international contests proved that she was prepared to compete at the top levels and that she had great potential for more success.

Public Recognition and Media Attention Simone's outstanding performances and accomplishments brought her a great deal of public and media attention. Due to her performance in senior events, she became more well-known and admired by the media and fans alike as a budding gymnastics star. The fact that Simone's skills and talents were widely acknowledged speaks to her influence on the sport.

SETTING UP FOR FUTURE ACHIEVEMENT

Ongoing Education and Training Simone kept her attention on her training and growth after her breakout performances. Her continued success as a top gymnast was largely dependent on her dedication to honing her routines, developing her talents, and getting ready for contests. Simone's continuous success can be attributed in large part to her commitment to her training and her quest for perfection.

 Naming New Objectives Simone's breakthrough accomplishments and senior debut laid the groundwork for her future ambitions. Her accomplishments gave her a solid platform on which to build her career as a gymnast. Setting and achieving new objectives was a crucial part of Simone's continuous development into one of the best gymnasts of all time.

Simone Biles's career underwent a sea change after her breakthrough performances and senior debut. She became recognized as a top gymnast and laid the foundation for her future success thanks to her outstanding performances in national and international competitions. Simone's incredible path from a rising star to a famous figure in the gymnastics world was emphasized by her dominance in the sport, her commitment to training, and her influence on the sport.

Mary A.Clapp

WORLD CHAMPIONSHIPS 2013

In Simone Biles' career, the 2013 World Championships in Antwerp, Belgium, were a historic occasion. She made history with a number of firsts at this competition, which helped to establish her as a dominant force in international gymnastics. Important Achievements and Highlights Gold Medal for All Around At the 2013 World Championships, Simone Biles created history by taking home the "all-around gold medal. She became the first African American gymnast to win the all-around title at a World Championship, making this triumph very noteworthy. Her performance in the all-around competition demonstrated her extraordinary skill and versatility on all apparatuses, which included floor exercises, vaults, uneven bars, and balance beams.

Gold Medals for Vault and Floor Work Simone's outstanding achievement went beyond the competition's all-around division. She excelled in both the floor exercise and the vault, winning gold medals for her efforts. While her floor exercise routines were highlighted by artful choreography and high-flying tumbling passes, her vault routine showcased powerful and accurate execution. Her status as a great gymnast was strengthened by her achievements, which also demonstrated her versatility.

Bronze Medal for Balance Beam Simone won a bronze medal on the balancing beam in addition to her gold medals. This accomplishment demonstrated her balance and expertise on this difficult piece of equipment. Simone's performance on the balancing beam was impressive despite the fierce competition, and it helped her win the tournament as a whole.

EVALUATION OF PERFORMANCE

Performance and Accuracy Simone's execution and accuracy during her performances at the 2013 World Championships were noteworthy. She distinguished herself from other gymnasts with her extraordinary accuracy and grace when executing difficult tasks. Her attention to detail in every routine demonstrated her commitment to training and planning.

Originality and Challenge Simone pushed the limits of gymnastics routines with her high difficulty and inventive aspects in her performances. She showed off her technical mastery and inventiveness by including difficult new talents into her performances. She became known as a top gymnast, and her performance at the championships was largely due to her inventiveness.

EFFECT ON PROFESSION

Achieving Global Notoriety For Simone Biles, the 2013 World Championships marked a sea change and made her a household name in the world of gymnastics. Her performance at this competition brought her widespread notoriety and cemented her place among the best players in the sport. Her increasing notoriety and chances for the future were facilitated by her performance at the World Championships.

Creating the Conditions for Future Achievement Simone's progress in gymnastics has been paved by the accolades and victories she earned at the 2013 World Championships. Her performance at these championships laid the groundwork for her later successes at national and international competitions and showed promise for future accomplishments.

A significant turning point in Simone Biles' career occurred at the 2013 World Championships in Antwerp, which catapulted her to stardom in the world of international gymnastics. Her accomplishments, which included bronze medals on the balance beam, vault, and all-around competitions in addition to gold medals in the floor exercise and vault, demonstrated her extraordinary talent and adaptability.

Simone's triumph in this tournament cemented her as a top gymnast and paved the way for her ongoing success and prominence in the gymnastics community. Improving Her Performance in Gymnastics After the 2013 World Championships, Simone Biles' career took off, and she quickly became recognized as the sport's dominant force thanks to a string of noteworthy successes. Her reputation as one of the sport's most formidable competitors was cemented by her outstanding performances, creative routines, and steady success.

Mary A.Clapp

Persistent Domination in Contests 2014–2015 U.S. National Championships In 2014 and 2015, Simone Biles maintained her success at the U.S. National Championships. She won the all-around competition in both years, solidifying her place as the top gymnast in the country. She also took home gold in the vault, floor exercise, and balancing beam competitions in 2014, and she did it again in 2015. Her ability to continuously execute at the highest level was demonstrated by her dominance at these national meets.

World Cups (in 2014 and 2015) In 2014 and 2015, Simone maintained her success on the international scene at the World Championships. She took home gold in all four apparatus categories at the 2014 Nanning, China, Olympics: vault, floor exercise, balancing beam, and all-around. Her remarkable achievement in these championships cemented her status as one of the best gymnasts in the history of the sport. Simone demonstrated her consistency and unwavering performance in 2015 as she won the all-around title and the gold in vault, floor exercise, and balance beam at the World Championships in Glasgow, Scotland.

Novelties and Distinctive Abilities Distinct Practices and Abilities Simone Biles' routines were notable for their inventive components and high level of difficulty. The "Biles" on floor exercise, which is a double layout with a half twist, and the "Biles" on vault, which is a handspring double front with a half twist, are two of the new skills and combinations she presented. Her trademark routines not only showcased her technical skill but also raised the bar for gymnastics.

Effect on Technique in Gymnastics The evolution of gymnastics routines and methods was impacted by Simone's ability to perform intricate routines with grace and accuracy. Other gymnasts were motivated to stretch their boundaries and add new components to their performances by her inventive skills and difficult routines. Within the sport of gymnastics, Simone's innovations and improvements to technique were generally acknowledged and appreciated.

Public Recognition and the Media International Notoriety Simone's accomplishments in gymnastics brought her widespread acclaim and substantial media coverage. Her accomplishments were extensively reported by the sports media, and she rose to prominence in the gymnastics community all around the world. Beyond the gymnastics world, young athletes from a variety of disciplines looked up to Simone as an inspiration and role model.

Promotions and Public Events Simone made several public appearances and endorsements as her notoriety grew. She started to become in demand as a spokesman for many companies and attended prestigious events, which increased her exposure and influence even more. Her established standing as a prominent figure in sports was facilitated by her public demeanor and media presence.

Inputs into the Success of the Team Top Team USA Simone Biles was instrumental in helping Team USA win a number of international tournaments. Her contributions to team events were crucial to the squad's gold medals at the Olympic Games and the World Championships. Simone's status as a pivotal athlete in American gymnastics was underlined by her leadership and contributions to the team's victory.

 Promoting Team Spirit Simone's perseverance and accomplishments motivated her teammates and strengthened Team USA's unity as a whole. Her presence and performance inspired a strong sense of teamwork among her fellow gymnasts and set a high bar for them. The group accomplishments of Team USA demonstrated Simone's impact and solidified her position as a major player in the sport.

 Legacy and Significance Gymnastics Redefined Beyond her personal accomplishments, Simone Biles has had a significant influence on gymnastics. Her ground-breaking routines, outstanding performances, and leadership have completely changed the sport and established new standards for upcoming generations. Simone's influence on the development of gymnastics and her ability to motivate emerging talent define her legacy.

 Role modeling and mentoring In addition to being a well-known gymnast, Simone Biles has assumed the roles of mentor and role model. Young gymnasts and aspiring athletes find motivation in their accomplishments and successes. Through her activism and mentoring, Simone continues to affect gymnastics' future, even beyond her professional career. Gymnast Simone Biles's rise to prominence is a result of her tremendous talent, creative routines, and steady success.

Her standing as one of the most important athletes in the sport was cemented by her accomplishments in both national and international championships, her influence on gymnastics technique, and her widespread reputation. The future of gymnastics is being shaped and inspired by Simone's leadership qualities, pioneering legacy, and contributions to the sport.

CHAPTER 6: INNOVATIONS AND SKILLS

Simone Biles has had a significant impact on gymnastics with her ground-breaking inventions and remarkable abilities, which have raised the bar for the discipline. Gymnastics has greatly benefited from her ability to execute and create intricate routines, which has pushed the envelope of what is conceivable.

 Unique Abilities Biles (Vault) The "Biles" is a vaulted handspring double front that has a half twist. Because of the innovative way in which Simone Biles performed this technique, it bears her name. Her vault is among the hardest in gymnastics, showcasing her extraordinary strength and dexterity. It's a unique part of her vault routine since it calls for extreme height and control.

Floor Exercise: Biles The floor workout known as "Biles" consists of two layouts with a half twist. This tumbling pass is renowned for both its amazing execution and extreme difficulty. Simone sets a new benchmark for floor workout routines with her masterful and highly controlled execution of this talent. The Biles are praised for combining grace and intricacy.

Floor Exercise: Biles II The "Biles II" is an improved version of her initial floor technique that incorporates a double layout with a complete twist. This move highlights her creative approach to floor routines and demonstrates her accuracy in performing intricate parts.

On Beam, Biles With her abilities, Simone has also significantly improved the balancing beam. She has demonstrated her ability to blend challenge with balance and grace by introducing new elements and combinations that have set standards in beam routines.

Novel Approaches to Regular Composition Intricate Tumbling Moves The intricate tumbling passes in

Mary A.Clapp

Simone Biles' routines are among the most demanding in gymnastics. Frequently, her floor workout regimens incorporate several challenging exercises, such as the double-twisting double layout (DTDL) and the double-twisting double backflip (DTY). These components accentuate her extraordinary strength and skill.

Decorative Aspects Simone's routines are renowned for their artistic expressiveness in addition to their technical prowess. Her floor workouts frequently feature choreography that enhances the overall performance and goes well with her tumbling passes. Her ability to combine artistic components with technical challenges has raised the bar for standard composition.

Effect on Athletics Establishing New Guidelines The possibilities in gymnastics have been broadened by Simone Biles' inventions and prowess. Her proficiency in performing extremely difficult routines has elevated the standard for gymnasts all around the world. Her introduction of skills and routines has influenced the direction of gymnastics methods and routines, setting standards for other athletes.

Mary A.Clapp

Sparking Originality Other gymnasts have been motivated to experiment with new components and push the boundaries of their routines by Simone's success. Her impact may be seen in the growing number of gymnasts who use creative aspects and extremely difficult abilities in their routines. Beyond just her personal accomplishments, Simone has influenced gymnastics as a whole.

Acknowledgment and Praise About Her Named Skills Given Simone Biles' influence on the sport, a number of her characteristic moves have been named after her. Her achievements and inventions are recognized by the gymnastics world, which is a testimonial to her skill. In gymnastics, the "Biles" and other things bearing her name have left a lasting impression.

Honors and Recognitions Simone has won multiple honors and recognitions for her achievements, including medals from the Olympics and World Championships. Her gymnastics accomplishments are acknowledged for their difficulty as well as their role in the development of the sport. The ideas and abilities of Simone Biles have permanently changed gymnastics. Her innovative routines and intricate talents have completely changed the sport, raising the bar on complexity and execution.

Beyond her accomplishments, Simone's influence will continue to shape gymnastics going forward and inspire new generations of athletes. Her outstanding accomplishments and ongoing influence have solidified her reputation as a gymnastics trailblazer. The Qualities That Set Simon Apart Throughout her gymnastics career, Simone Biles has demonstrated a number of extraordinary abilities that have raised the bar for the sport. She is considered one of the greatest gymnasts of all time because of these abilities, which are distinguished by their difficulty, precision, and inventiveness.

Skills from the Vault Biles (Vault) The "Biles" is an impressively controlled and high-handspring double front with a half twist. Because of her innovative use of it, Simone Biles is honored in the name of this skill. The height, speed, and exact landing that are necessary for the vault add to Its Intricacy. Simone's vault is a signature move in her gymnastics arsenal because of her exceptional execution of it.

Amanar (Vault) In addition, Simone does the Amanar, a 2.5 twist handspring. Although she did not create the vault, the way she executed it is remarkable for its strength and accuracy. Simone possesses extraordinary skill in delivering the necessary combination of speed, height, and rotation to defeat the Amanar.

 Skills for Floor Exercises Floor Exercise: Biles The floor workout known as "Biles" consists of two layouts with a half twist. This high-flying execution and the difficulty of the falling pass are well known. Simone's display of this talent is praised for fusing intricate gymnastics with a beautiful presentation.

 Floor Exercise: Biles II An upgraded version of her initial floor pass, the "Biles II, has a double layout with a full twist. This component shows off her ability to execute high-challenge talents precisely while adding another level of difficulty to her routine.

 Equilibrium Beam Proficiencies On Beam, Biles In her balancing beam performance, Simone has included a number of new features, including intricate dismounts and unusual skill combinations. She frequently incorporates creative aspects into her beam performances to show off her balance, control, and inventiveness.

SKILLS FOR UNEVEN BARS

Regular Innovations by Biles Although Simone's floor and vault routines have garnered her the most attention, her uneven bar routines also highlight her talent and originality. Her overall gymnastics prowess is enhanced by her ability to execute intricate release routines and transitions with precision and grace.

Technical and Creative Expertise Difficulty with Grace in Balance The combination of technical challenge and creative execution characterizes Simone's routines. Her unique ability to combine difficult abilities into emotive and flowing routines makes her stand out from other gymnasts. Every performance is painstakingly planned to accentuate her best qualities and uphold her high caliber of artistic ability.

Precision and ConsistencySimone's success depends heavily on how consistently and precisely she uses her skills. Her skill, dedication, and training are evident in her ability to execute challenging tasks with few mistakes and to perform at a high level on several apparatuses.

Legacy and Significance Establishing New Guidelines In gymnastics, Simone Biles's abilities have raised the bar and influenced choreography and performance. Her creative components and extremely challenging routines have been ingrained in the sport, encouraging gymnasts everywhere to challenge the limits of their own routines.

Model for Inspiration Because of her proficiency with these techniques, Simone is now regarded as an idol in gymnastics. Aspiring gymnasts might take inspiration from her accomplishments and distinguishing skills, which show what can be accomplished with remarkable talent and devotion. The talents that characterize Simone Biles—from her ground-breaking vaults to her creative floor exercise passes—showcase her unmatched ability and impact in the gymnastics community.

Her ability to blend creative expression with technical challenges has revolutionized the sport and left a lasting legacy. As one of the greatest athletes in gymnastics history, Simone's accomplishments will no doubt inspire upcoming generations of gymnasts.

HOW SHE DEFINED HARDNESS IN THE GYM

By raising the bar for what is deemed achievable in the sport and redefining difficulty standards, Simone Biles has completely changed the landscape of gymnastics. Her efforts have elevated the bar for performance excellence and technical complexity, creating new standards for upcoming generations.

Innovating New Proficiencies Vault Innovations A few high-difficulty vaults, such as the Biles (a handspring double front with a half twist) and the Amanar (a handspring with a 2.5 twist), were invented and developed by Simone Biles. It takes great strength, height, and accuracy to operate these vaults. The Biles in particular, who displayed abilities never before seen in the sport of vaulting, perfectly captures the tremendous difficulties she introduced to the sport.

Passes for Floor Exercises The Biles, a double layout with a half twist, and the Biles II, a double layout with a complete twist, are two of the ways that Biles contribute to floor workout regimens. These passes are not only difficult, but they are also performed with such grace and force that they have raised the bar for what is thought to be possible during floor workouts. Her creative passes have altered how routines are put together and redefined the degree of difficulty for tumbling passes.

Increasing the Regular Complexity High-Difficulty Element Integration Several extremely challenging components are frequently combined into a single performance in Simone's routines. Her floor exercise performances, for example, combine technical difficulties with artistic expression through a combination of sophisticated choreography and demanding tumbling passes. Her capacity to uphold excellent performance standards in a variety of gymnastics-related domains is demonstrated by this integration of elements.

Mary A.Clapp

Precision and Consistency Redefining difficulty largely depends on how consistently Simone executes these challenging parts. Her precision and low error rate in executing intricate talents have raised the bar for performance dependability. This regularity in extremely challenging routines highlights the fact that mastering certain skills is just as important as having the skills themselves.

EFFECT ON EVALUATION AND ASSESSMENT

Affecting Difficulty Ratings Gymnasts now assess and appraise difficulty differently as a result of Simone's introduction of new talents and components of greater complexity. Her results have shown that the sport can accept and even reward more complexity, which has led to revisions in the scoring criteria and an increased focus on scoring difficulty.

Establishing New Guidelines Because of Simone's contributions to gymnastics, new standards for difficulty have been set, and as a result, gymnasts' approaches to their routines have changed. Her standards have inspired players to think outside the box and add more challenging components to their performances, which will help to shape the sport's future.

Inspirational Guidance Promoting Creativity Because of Simone's achievement, gymnasts all over the world are now motivated to push themselves and create new possibilities for their routines. Her ability to reinterpret difficulties has inspired other athletes to add difficult routines and creative components, furthering gymnastics' continuous development.

Assigning Priorities All levels of gymnasts now have higher expectations because of Simone's level of difficulty. Athletes and coaches now understand that reaching a high degree of difficulty is necessary for success, and they work hard to match or go beyond Simone's expectations. Her impact on the gymnastics world is not limited to her personal performances.

LEGACY AND IMPLICATIONS FOR THE FUTURE

Persistent Impact The influence of Simone Biles on gymnastics difficulty is long-lasting and significant. Her efforts have created a new paradigm for the sport, in addition to redefining what is achievable. Gymnastics will be influenced by the techniques she developed and introduced for years to come.

Building the Next Generation Gymnastics' future will be shaped by Simone's redefined difficulty, which will serve as a guide for upcoming generations of gymnasts striving for perfection. Her inventions have raised the standard for technical and artistic performance, motivating athletes in the future to reach new heights and further redefine their sport.

Simone Biles's innovative abilities, seamless incorporation of intricate aspects, and unwavering dedication to performance have completely changed the level of difficulty in gymnastics. Her impact has changed the sport, encouraging athletes all around the world and establishing new benchmarks. Simone's outstanding contributions to gymnastics, which enhanced the sport's difficulty and artistry and shaped its future, leave a lasting legacy.

CHAPTER 7: DOMINANCE ON THE WORLD STAGE

Simone Biles's unmatched achievements and unwavering success in international gymnastics events define her dominance on the global stage. Her accomplishments have cemented her status as one of the best gymnasts of all time and established a new benchmark for performance in the sport.

Notable Accomplishments World Championships in 2013 At the 2013 World Championships in Antwerp, Belgium, Simone Biles first made a big impression on the international scene. She became the first African American gymnast to win the all-around championship. In addition, she won gold in the floor and vault exercises and a bronze in the balancing beam competition. These triumphs showed off her adaptability and technical skill on a variety of equipment.

World Championships in 2014 Simone Biles displayed her dominance once again during the 2014 World Championships in Nanning, China. In the four events—all-around, vault, floor exercise, and balancing beam—she took home gold medals. Her remarkable skill and consistency were demonstrated by her ability to excel in every apparatus, solidifying her status as one of the top gymnasts in the world.

World Championships in 2015 At the 2015 World Championships in Glasgow, Scotland, Simone Biles won gold in the vault, floor exercise, balance beam, and all-around events. She continued her unbeaten run in the World Championships and cemented her position as a dominant force in international gymnastics with her precise and inventive performance.

Rio Olympics 2016 The 2016 Rio Olympics performance by Simone marked a turning point in her career. In addition to a bronze medal on the balance beam, she took home four gold medals: all-around, vault, floor exercise, and team. Her outstanding talent and training were evident in her dominance during the Olympics, and she played a crucial role in Team USA's victory.

World Championships in 2017 Simone Biles extended her winning streak in the 2017 World Championships in Montreal, Canada, where she won gold in the vault, floor exercise, and all-around competitions. Her accomplishments proved that she could continue to be one of the best athletes in the sport for an extended period of time.

Tokyo Olympics 2021 Simone Biles competed at the 2021 Tokyo Olympics despite facing severe personal obstacles. With a bronze medal on the balancing beam, she made a spectacular return and helped the American team to victory overall. Her choice to put her mental health first and perform well under duress demonstrated her fortitude and dedication to the game.

Advantage over Competition Expertise in Technology Simone Biles's technical proficiency is what defines her dominance. Some of the most challenging components in gymnastics history are included in her routines, which are completed with calm and precision. Her competitive advantage stems from her ability to think outside the box and execute tasks consistently.

Mental and Physical Power A major contributing aspect to Simone's dominance is her mental toughness and combination of physical strength and training. Her remarkable mental toughness is demonstrated by her capacity to perform well under duress and bounce back from failures, which enables her to compete at her best in high-stakes situations.

Legacy and Influence Motivation for Sportspeople Gymnasts and athletes in a variety of disciplines have been motivated by Simone Biles's success on the international scene. Her accomplishments and tenacity serve as an inspiration for aspiring athletes, showing the heights that may be attained through commitment and diligence.

Mary A.Clapp

Establishing New Guidelines Because of Simone's supremacy, gymnastics routine design and execution have changed significantly. Her efforts have elevated the bar for difficulty and execution, influencing the sport's future and pushing other gymnasts to improve their routines. Simone Biles has dominated the world stage thanks to her extraordinary accomplishments, technical prowess, and capacity for high-pressure performance.

Her accomplishments in global events, including the Olympic Games and the World Championships, have cemented her place as one of the all-time greatest gymnasts. Beyond her professional career, Simone has inspired upcoming generations of athletes and set new benchmarks in gymnastics.

THE PATH TO RIO

Simone Biles underwent a time of rigorous training, calculated planning, and incredible accomplishments leading up to the 2016 Rio Olympics. Her relentless gymnastics dominance, intense training regimen, and important events that paved the way for her Olympic glory defined her journey to Rio. Important Turning Points

 World Championships in 2015 On Simone Biles' journey to the Rio Olympics, the 2015 World Championships in Glasgow, Scotland, was a critical turning point. She took home gold in the vault, floor exercise, balance beam, and all-around events. Her performance proved that she was ready for the next Olympics and cemented her place as the best gymnast in the world. Her preparation for the Olympics greatly benefited from the energy and confidence this achievement gave her.

U.S. National Championships: Simone Biles participated in the U.S. competition prior to Rio. National Titles in the years 2015 and 2016. She took home gold in many apparatuses and the all-around crown in both years. Her dominance and consistency in national tournaments were demonstrated by these performances, solidifying her place as one of the top contenders for the Olympics.

Mary A.Clapp

Olympic Trials One of the most important stops on Simone Biles' path to Rio was the U.S. Olympic Trials in July of 2016. She gave an outstanding performance, taking home the all-around title and earning a spot on the U.S. Olympic squad competing in gymnastics. Her preparation and expertise were evident in her impressive trial performances, which paved the way for her Olympic glory.

 Get Ready and Get Trained Strong Training Plan Simone Biles underwent a rigorous training program in order to get ready for the Olympics in Rio. Her training aimed to strengthen her body, improve her mental toughness, and refine her routines. The demanding program was created to guarantee optimal performance and preparedness for the intensely competitive Olympic setting.

 Psychological Readiness Simone worked on her mental preparedness in addition to her physical training. These included stress-reduction, concentration, and motivation-boosting techniques. Her capacity to perform well under the intense scrutiny and strain of the Olympic

Mary A.Clapp

Games was largely dependent on her mental toughness.

DIFFICULTIES AND GETTING PAST BARRIERS
INJURY CONCERNS

Simone had some physical worries on the way to Rio, including small problems with her ankle and shoulder. She performed well and kept to her training regimen in spite of these obstacles. Her training for the Olympics was greatly aided by her tenacity and capacity to bounce back from physical setbacks.

School and Gymnastics in Balance Simone also had to juggle her school obligations with gymnastics training. It was difficult for her to strike an appropriate balance between her demanding training schedule and her studies, but she did it in order to remain committed to her Olympic aspirations.

Accomplishments Before Rio Global Achievement Prior to the Olympics, Simone enjoyed success on a global scale by winning a number of contests, such as the 2015 World Championships and the 2016 AT&T American Cup. Her flawless success at these competitions proved that she was prepared and raised hopes for her Olympic performance.

Group Structure Important components of Simone's preparation were her relationships with her teammates and her position on the U.S. gymnastics team. Attaining success as a team at the Olympics required fostering good team relationships and mutual support. Simone Biles paved the way to the 2016 Rio Olympics with her remarkable performances, intense training, and unwavering devotion.

Her remarkable achievements in Rio were made possible by her capacity to overcome obstacles, her ability to succeed in important competitions, and her rigorous training. Simone's road to the Olympics is a perfect example of her passion for gymnastics and her resolve to compete at the highest level worldwide.

GETTING READY FOR THE OLYMPICS 2016

Simone Biles' meticulously organized and carried out Olympic preparation for the 2016 Rio Games was a testament to her passion and devotion to gymnastics excellence. A combination of rigorous training, calculated planning, and inner fortitude went into this preparation.

Exercise Schedule Motivation through Exercise An essential component of Simone Biles' training was her physical conditioning. Among her training exercises were: "Strength Training": concentrating on developing the strength required to do highly challenging skills accurately. Exercises for Flexibility: These are crucial for carrying out intricate routines and preserving movement flexibility.

Technical Drills: Focusing on refining routines like vaults, floor exercises, uneven bars, and balance beams. Perfect Routine Simone practiced a lot, which allowed her routines to be consistently improved. Her instruction centered on: "Skill Execution": To guarantee flawless performance during competitions, high-difficulty skills must be practiced and perfected.

Mary A.Clapp

Routine Choreography: Including intricate details into routines without sacrificing flow or artistic expression. Simulated Performances: Practicing in a competitive environment to get ready for the demands of the Olympic arena.

 Mental Readiness Resilience in the Mind Simone Biles needed to mentally prepare herself in order to withstand the strain of the Olympics. This included: Visualization Techniques: Visualizing successful performances and practicing routines with mental images.

Stress Management: Strategies for controlling anxiousness before competitions and staying focused when things get tough. Goal Setting: Clearly defining your goals and staying inspired during the planning stage. Support Systems

 Simone was dependent on a network of allies that comprised: Coaching Staff: offering direction, criticism, and modifications to her training schedule. Sports psychologists: Offering resilience training and mental tactics assistance. Family and Friends: Providing her with moral support and inspiration along the way.

Important Contests U.S. National Championships: The performances Simone gave at the U.S. The 2015 and 2016 National Championships were crucial. Her triumphs in these competitions proved that she was prepared and cemented her place among the top candidates for the Olympics.

Olympic Trials A crucial aspect of her preparation took place in July 2016 during the U.S. Olympic Trials. Prior to the Olympics, Simone's outstanding performance at the trials guaranteed her spot on the U.S. gymnastics squad and displayed her best form.

Overcoming Obstacles Injuries Control Simone sustained minor ailments during her preparation, including problems with her ankle and shoulder. Involved in efficient injury management: Medical Treatment: Getting the right attention and recuperation to make a full recovery. Adjusting Training: She changed her training schedule to prevent aggravating her injuries while keeping her level of performance.

Combining Accountabilities Simone had to manage her demanding training schedule in addition to her personal and academic obligations. Using time management techniques helped her stay focused and make sure that every detail of her preparation was taken care of.

Last-Minute Planning Relaxation and Taping Simone's training changed in the last several weeks before the Olympics, with an emphasis on tapering: Lowering Training Intensity: Giving her body more time to heal and reach its best for the Olympics. Mental Focus: finalizing regular details and honing mental tactics.

Group Structure The team's overall performance depended heavily on her ability to establish good team dynamics and cultivate favorable relationships with her teammates. The cohesiveness and morale of the U.S. gymnastics team were enhanced by Simone's leadership role and her encouragement of her teammates.

Simone Biles used a multifaceted method to prepare for the 2016 Rio Olympics, which included intense physical training, mental preparation, and skillful problem-solving. Her outstanding performance at the Olympics was largely due to her commitment to honing her talents as well as to strategic preparation and support networks. Simone's careful planning is a testament to her dedication to attaining success and her willingness to succeed globally.

Team USA and What's Possible In addition to being a major component of the larger Team USA gymnastics program, Simone Biles' desire for perfection led her to the 2016 Rio Olympics. Because of the team's remarkable potential and track record of success, there were high hopes for Team USA. The Achievements and Past of Team USA Prior Accomplishments International competition achievement is a longstanding accomplishment for Team USA Gymnastics.

Among the group's accomplishments are: Olympic Gold Medals: The "Magnificent Seven" in 1996 and the "Final Five" in 2016 are two noteworthy triumphs. World Championships: Team USA has demonstrated its dominance in gymnastics on a worldwide scale by routinely performing well at the World Championships.

Excellence Legacy Expectations for the 2016 Rio Olympics were high due to the legacy of Team USA. Athletes were expected to match or above this standard of excellence due to the team's track record of success.

Mary A.Clapp

Simone Biles and her colleagues knew they had an obligation to maintain this custom.

The Olympic Team of 2016 Makeup of the Team 2016 U.S. Women's Gymnastics Team members were: Simone Biles: well-known for her remarkable talent and commanding stage presence. Gabby Douglas: The Olympic all-around champion from 2012, who brings success from the past and experience. Aly Raisman is a talented performer with a solid resume who is reliable and skilled. Laurene Hernandez is a budding talent renowned for her creative routines and exuberant live shows. Madison Kocian is well-known for her versatility and skill with uneven bars.

Group Structure The team's dynamics and chemistry were essential to its success. The team members cooperated, gave each other support, and shared tasks in order to accomplish their objectives. The leadership and uplifting influence of Simone Biles were essential in creating a motivated and cohesive team atmosphere.

Pressure and Expectations Excellent Work Standards Expectations for Team USA were especially high because of the team's heritage and the presence of strong athletes: Gold Medal Contenders: The group was anticipated to be among the front-runners for the team competition's gold medal.

Individual Success: It was believed that Simone Biles and her teammates would do well on their own, with multiple gymnasts predicted to contend for gold in the individual apparatus and all-around competitions. Public and Media Attention The public's and media's rigorous scrutiny increased the pressure. Extensive media attention accompanied the high expectations, showcasing Team USA's potential as well as its difficulties; the participants had to balance this pressure with their performance.

Fulfilling Aspirations Group Achievement At the Rio Olympics in 2016, Team USA lived up to their lofty expectations by taking home the gold medal as a team. Their show was distinguished by superb routines, amazing technique, and a strong sense of teamwork. This triumph fulfilled the great expectations that were put on Team USA and confirmed their dominance in gymnastics.

Personal Accomplishments Particularly, Simone Biles's performances went above and beyond what was anticipated. Gold Medals: She took home four golds in the vault, floor exercise, team, and all-around competitions, plus one bronze in the balancing beam competition.

Historic Performance: Her accomplishments raised the bar for gymnastics and greatly aided the team's success. The remarkable skill of its individuals and the team's distinguished past influenced the expectations surrounding Team USA at the 2016 Rio Olympics. These were not only reached, but beyond, by Simone Biles and her teammates, who gave a remarkable and historic performance. Their accomplishments emphasized Team USA's might and solidified their reputation in the gymnastics community.

Mary A.Clapp

CHAPTER 8: 2016 RIO OLYMPICS

Gymnastics history and Simone Biles's career both underwent significant changes during the 2016 Rio Olympics. These games, which took place in Rio de Janeiro, Brazil, highlighted Team USA's strength and Simone's incredible talent, leading to a number of outstanding performances. Summary of Simone Biles's Act Group Contest Gold Medal: In the team competition, Madison Kocian, Laurie Hernandez, Aly Raisman, Simone Biles, and Gabby Douglas from Team USA took first place. There was remarkable skill, accuracy, and teamwork in the team's performance. Their triumph demonstrated the strength of their unity and confirmed Team USA's supremacy in gymnastics.

Single Occurrences All-Around: Simone Biles performed flawlessly on every apparatus to win the gold medal in the all-around category. Her routines demonstrated extreme difficulty, flawless technique, and artistic flair, securing her place as the world's best gymnast. Vault: Simone's performance on the vault earned her another gold medal. The highlight of the competition was her performance of the Biles (handspring double front with a half twist), which showed off her strength and dexterity.

Floor activity: Simone won her third gold medal in this activity. Her performance, which featured the Biles (double layout with a half twist) and the Biles II (double layout with a full twist), was praised for its unique blend of beautiful presentation and challenging tumbling passes. Balance Beam: Simone won a bronze medal for her performance on the balance beam. Her routine, which displayed her balance, poise, and technical prowess, was impressive, even if it wasn't as dominant as her prior performances.

 Important Times Classic Rituals Simone Biles's technical complexity and flawless execution were highlights of her Olympic routines in Rio. Important times include: Floor dance: Her floor dance, which included creative tumbling passes, was praised widely for its intricate choreography and aerial components. Vault Performance: One of the most difficult and impressive vaults in the competition, the Biles vault, was performed with remarkable height and control.

Impact on Emotions and Inspiration Simone gave performances that were emotionally stirring in addition to being technically amazing. Millions were inspired by her accomplishment, which also brought attention to the tenacity and commitment needed to become the best gymnast in the world.

 Strategy and Team Dynamics Unity and Assistance Strong team dynamics contributed to Team USA's victory as well. The participants' encouragement of one another during each exercise fostered a cooperative and upbeat atmosphere that improved their performance as a whole.

Training and Getting Ready The success of the team was largely dependent on their preparation, which was overseen by coaches like Marta Karolyi and her staff. The participants were certain to be in top form for the Olympics, thanks to their intense training regimen and careful preparation.

Mary A.Clapp

Public and Media Attention Global Acknowledgment**
The performances by Simone Biles attracted a lot of
praise and media attention. Her accomplishments were
warmly hailed and helped gymnastics gain more
acceptance as a prominent sport.

Importance and Legacy Simone's reputation as one of
the greatest gymnasts of all time was solidified by her
performance at the Olympics in Rio. Her
accomplishments inspired upcoming generations of
competitors and set new benchmarks in the sport.
Gymnast Simone Biles and Team USA made history at
the 2016 Rio Olympics.

With her incredible achievements, which included
multiple gold medals and a bronze, Simone cemented
her legacy in gymnastics history and demonstrated her
unmatched brilliance. The Games brought to light the
power, talent, and camaraderie that characterized Team
USA's accomplishments and created an enduring
impression on the sport.

MEDALS AND HISTORIC PERFORMANCES

The 2016 Rio Olympics saw Simone Biles give absolutely spectacular performances, breaking gymnastics records and winning a ton of medals in a variety of events. Her supremacy and mastery of technique were two of the Games' greatest moments.

Historical Acts Competition All Around Gold Medal: With a final score of 62.198, Simone Biles took home the gold in the all-around competition. Her performance stood out for its extreme difficulty and faultless execution on the balancing beam, vault, uneven bars, and floor exercise. With this triumph, she established herself as the world's finest all-around gymnast and showcased her extensive skill set and adaptability.

Vault-Gold Medal: With a cumulative score of 15.966, Simone Biles demonstrated exceptional vaulting performance to earn gold. One of the hardest vaults ever attempted in a competition was the Biles, a handspring double front with a half twist that she did throughout her performance. Her completion of her vault demonstrated remarkable dexterity and height.

Active Floor Work-Gold Medal: With a score of 15.966 in the floor exercise, Biles took first place. She performed the Biles (a half-twisted double layout) and the Biles II (a full-twisted double configuration) in her routine. The routine's exquisite choreography, immaculate execution, and daring tumbling passes won it praise.

 Equilibrium Beam-Bronze Medal: Simone's score of 15.433 on the balancing beam earned her a bronze medal. Despite not having the best score, her routine showed off her grace, balance, and technical proficiency. Even though it wasn't as strong as her previous events, her performance on the balancing beam demonstrated her extraordinary skills.

 Awards and Accomplishments Medals of Gold-Team Competition: A key member of the American squad that took home the gold in the team competition was Simone Biles. Her efforts on each of the four apparatuses contributed to Team USA's overall success and helped to seal the team's triumph. All-Around: One of the highlights of Biles' Olympic career was her gold medal win in the all-around, which cemented her status as the world's best gymnast. Vault: Biles' creative and extremely challenging vaults earned her the gold medal in vault, creating a new benchmark for the competition. Floor Exercise: She further proved her supremacy in gymnastics with her gold medal in floor exercise, which was a tribute to her artistic presentation and tumbling abilities.

Medal of Bronze-Balance Beam: Simone Biles' triumph in the bronze medal round on the balance beam was noteworthy as it demonstrated her capacity to execute well under duress, even in the face of fierce opposition. Her total success was enhanced by the medal, which also demonstrated her versatility.

Legacy and Significance Establishing New Guidelines Gymnastics records were set by Simone Biles's performances at the Rio Olympics. Her extremely challenging routines and faultless performance raised the bar for aspiring gymnasts and had an impact on the development of the sport.

Mary A.Clapp

Motivating Next Generations The accomplishments of Biles inspired young athletes everywhere. Her accomplishment inspired the next generation to push boundaries and strive for greatness by showcasing the potential in gymnastics. The 2016 Rio Olympics saw Simone Biles deliver incredible performances and take home medals, which made history in the sport of gymnastics.

Her remarkable talent and dominance in the sport were highlighted by her gold medals in the floor exercise, vault, and all-around, as well as her bronze in the balancing beam. Her reputation as one of the best gymnasts of all time was cemented by these accomplishments, which also raised the bar for gymnastics brilliance.

A FOLLOW-UP TO OLYMPIC SUCCESS

In the wake of her incredible Rio Olympics triumph in 2016, Simone Biles underwent a great deal of personal and professional growth. Her Olympic achievement opened up new doors for her and came with obligations, problems, and chances. Direct Effect Notice to the Public and Media The public was impressed by Simone Biles's accomplishments in Rio, and she received extensive media coverage. She became well-known as a representation of gymnastics brilliance.

Among the highlights of the strong media attention were: Interviews and Appearances: Simone shared her experiences and celebrated her achievements on a number of talk programs, interviews, and media events. Public Recognition: She was recognized for her achievements in athletics and her role as an inspiration by a number of organizations and institutions with awards, honors, and accolades.

 Partnerships and Endorsements The Olympic success of Simone Biles brought her a plethora of endorsement deals and partnerships. Businesses and brands aspired to be associated with her prominent achievements, which resulted in: Brand Partnerships: Simone has agreements with Procter & Gamble, Nike, and Visa, among other well-known companies. These collaborations included product endorsements, ads, and promotional campaigns. Financial options: She made a substantial rise in income thanks to the sponsorships and endorsements, which gave her stability and new options.

Professional Advancements Ongoing Career in Gymnastics After the Olympics in Rio, Simone Biles carried on with her gymnastics career, achieving a number of noteworthy milestones: 2017 World Championships: She won gold in the vault, floor exercise, and all-around events as she successfully defended her championship in Montreal. 2018 and Beyond: After a brief break from professional gymnastics, Simone went back to the sport, training for upcoming competitions and breaking records.

Participation in Additional Projects Following the Olympics, Simone worked on a number of non-gymnastics-related projects: Book Publications: She wrote books describing her life, career, and experiences, one of which was an autobiography. TV and Media: Simone's fame grew outside gymnastics when she made appearances in reality TV and dance competitions.

 Impact on the Individual and Society Action and Support Simone Biles promoted significant causes using her platform: Mental Health Awareness: She encouraged people to seek treatment by speaking candidly about mental health issues. Her willingness to share personal experiences with others de-stigmatized mental health conditions. Support for Survivors: Simone was outspoken in her advocacy for victims of abuse and in her discussion of matters pertaining to the security and welfare of athletes.

Inspiration and Role Model Simone Biles rose to prominence as a global role model for youth athletes and people in general. Inspiration: Numerous people were motivated to follow their aspirations and overcome challenges by her accomplishments and tenacity. Mentorship: Simone participated in outreach and mentoring initiatives, fostering perseverance and good sportsmanshlp In young gymnasls.

 Difficulties and Modifications Controlling Anticipations Following her Olympic accomplishment, Simone faced enormous expectations, which brought challenges: Pressure and Scrutiny: Simone had to balance the demands of the public and media on her while keeping her performance standards high. Managing Personal and Professional Life: It took considerable planning to strike a balance between her obligations in her personal life and her health.

Health and Mental Welfare Preserving one's physical and mental well-being remained a top concern. Injury Management: Simone took care of any physical problems or injuries to make sure she could compete successfully moving forward. Mental Health: Maintaining her mental well-being was essential to juggling the demands of a prominent profession.

Following Simone Biles's gold medal in the Rio Olympics in 2016, a number of important developments and opportunities emerged. Her significance within and outside of the sport was demonstrated by her enlarged media presence, advocacy efforts, and ongoing gymnastics career. Notwithstanding the difficulties, Simone's post-Olympic career has been distinguished

by her ongoing successes, development as a person,
and significant stature in the public eye.

CHAPTER 9: WORLD CHAMPIONSHIP EXCELLENCE

Simone Biles' status as one of the best gymnasts of all time has been cemented by her accomplishments at the World Championships. Her performance at these esteemed competitions is a testament to her extraordinary talent, reliability, and love for the game.

World Championships 2013, held in Antwerp, Belgium Innovative Display- Gold Medals: Simone Biles took home the gold in the vault, floor exercise, balance beam, and all-around competitions. Impact: She became a rising gymnastics sensation after this tournament, which was also her first significant international triumph. Her performances stood out for their exceptional dexterity and accuracy.

World Championships 2014 (Nanning, China) Dominance - Gold Medals: Simone repeated her triumph from the previous year by winning gold in the all-around, vault, floor exercise, and balancing beam events. Historic Achievement: She became the first female gymnast to win back-to-back World Championship all-around titles in 1994 when she triumphed in the all-around. She gained notoriety for her ground-breaking routines and abilities. 2015 World Championships (Scotland's Glasgow)

Persistent Quality - Gold Medals: Simone Biles took home the gold in the vault, floor exercise, balance beam, and all-around competitions. Importance: This occasion demonstrated her reliability and supremacy over a number of years. Her Glasgow performance was crucial in generating interest in the 2016 Rio Olymplcs. She made a substantial contribution to Team USA's victory in the team competition as well.

Mary A.Clapp

Doha, Qatar: 2018 World Championships Go Back to Form- Gold Medals: Simone Biles returned with a bang, taking home gold in the vault, floor exercise, and all-around competitions. Recovery and Resilience: Her triumph at the 2018 World Championships proved that she was resilient and capable of getting back to her best after a hiatus. Her routines were praised for their artistic merit and superior technical skill.

World Championships in 2019 (Germany, Stuttgart) Trends of History- Gold Medals: Simone's victories in the vault, floor exercise, balancing beam, and all-around solidified her reputation as one of the top gymnasts. Record-Breaking Achievements: She broke the previous record for the most gold medals earned at these championships to become the most decorated gymnast in the history of the World Championships. Highlights of the competition were her creative skills, which included the Biles II on floor and the Yurchenko double pike on vault.

Legacy and Significance Difficulty and Innovation The gymnastics world has witnessed routines at the World Championships by Simone Biles that continuously push the envelope. Her proficiency with challenging techniques has raised the bar for the sport.

Influence and Motivation The gymnasts of the future have been motivated by her accomplishments. In addition to impacting gymnastics' technical aspects, Simone's accomplishments have helped to increase the sport's visibility internationally. Simone Biles' outstanding ability and commitment are demonstrated by her success at the World Championships.

 Her unwavering success—which includes numerous gold medals and noteworthy accomplishments—has made her a pivotal figure in gymnastics. Her accomplishments have shaped the sport and motivated athletes throughout.

RECORD-BREAKING SUCCESS

 Numerous record-breaking accomplishments during Simone Biles' career attest to her outstanding talent and impact in gymnastics. Her feats have redefined what is possible in the sport and established new benchmarks. Comprehensive Titles International Titles - Consecutive Titles: In 2014 and 2015, Simone Biles won the World Championships' all-around competition, making history as the first female gymnast to do so. Her unmatched skill and consistency were on full display as she dominated these competitions.

The Most Complete World TitlesRecord: By 2019, Biles has amassed the most all-around medals ever won by a female gymnast at the World Championships—five overall. Her accomplishments in this area highlight her consistent proficiency and adaptability on all platforms.

 Awards and Medals Worlds' Most Gold Medals Record: With 19 gold medals overall as of 2019, Simone Biles owns the record for the most gold medals earned at the World Championships. This record demonstrates her years-long supremacy and reliability.

Highest Global Awards - Record: Including gold and other medals, Biles has won the most overall medals at the World Championships. Her total medal count exceeds historical highs, demonstrating her all-around prowess in a variety of sports.

New Developments and Proficiencies -Vault Innovations

The Biles: Simone debuted a brand-new vault that is a handspring double front with a half twist, called the Biles. This skill raises the bar in vaulting, as it is one of the hardest and riskiest vaults ever attempted.

The Yurchenko Double Pike: Biles executed the Yurchenko Double Pike vault in 2019, which was another first that pushed the limits of vaulting complexity.

Skills for Floor Exercise -The Biles II: One of the trickiest and most spectacular tumbling passes in gymnastics history, the 'Biles II' is a double layout with a full twist that was a part of Simone's floor exercise routine.

Olympic Accomplishments

' Rio Olympics 2016' - Most Gold Medals by a Female Gymnast at a Single Olympics: Simone Biles became the most decorated female gymnast in a single Olympic Games in 2016 when she won four gold medals in Rio.

Mary A.Clapp

She won gold in the vault, floor exercise, all-around, and team competitions.

Durability and Reliability

'Perpetual Domination' Over Multiple Championships': Biles has proven to be incredibly durable and consistent throughout her career, retaining her position as the top gymnast over numerous Olympic Games and World Championships. Her remarkable talent and commitment are demonstrated by her many years of top-notch performance.

Legacy and Influence

Taking Gymnastics Back

mpact on the Sport: Gymnastics norms have been redefined as a result of Simone Biles' record-breaking accomplishments. Her creative abilities, dependability, and caliber of performance have impacted the sport's development and motivated upcoming gymnast generations.

Athletes' Inspiration- Global Inspiration: Biles' accomplishments and records have elevated her to the status of a global gymnastics icon. Athletes all throughout the world have been motivated to push their own boundaries and pursue greatness by her achievements.

Gymnast Simone Biles has broken numerous records, which is a testament to her extraordinary talent, commitment, and influence. Her position as one of the best gymnasts of all time has been cemented by her several titles, creative abilities, and unwavering supremacy. Gymnastics will continue to be shaped and inspired by her accomplishments.

ESSENTIAL OUTCOMES AND THEIR IMPORTANCE

A number of significant performances throughout Simone Biles' career have had a significant influence on gymnastics. Her outstanding abilities were on full display throughout these performances, which also helped bring about important advancements and modifications in the sport.

Mary A.Clapp

World Championships 2013, held in Antwerp, Belgium

Highlights of Performance 'All-Around Gold': Biles elevated the bar for young gymnasts by winning her first gold medal in the all-around competition. Both judges and spectators were amazed by the technical difficulties and artistic execution of her performance.

'Gold Medals in Vault and Floor Exercise': Her highly skilled and creative routines were first showcased to the gymnastics community with her gold medals in both domains.

'Noteworthy'

'Breakthrough Achievement': With this competition, Simone became a major contender on the international scene and became recognized as a gymnastics emerging star. Foundation for Future Success: Her achievements paved the way for her to stay successful and have an impact on the sport going forward. World Championships 2014 (Nanning, China)

'Highlights of Performance' 'All-Around Gold: By successfully defending her title, Biles made history as the first female gymnast to win the World Championships' all-around competition twice in a row since 1994.

'Vault Gold': Showcased her creativity in the vault by introducing the 'Biles', a handspring double front with a half twist.

Noteworthy

'Historic Achievement': Her dominance and consistency were highlighted by her successive all-around titles, solidifying her place among the world's best gymnasts.

Innovation: The sport's technical difficulty advanced significantly with the debut of the 'Biles' vault.

2015 World Championships (Scotland's Glasgow)

'Highlights of Performance'- 'All-Around Gold': Biles achieved her third straight all-around championship, highlighting her consistency and adaptability.

'Floor Exercise Gold': She showcased her leadership skills in creative routines by performing the **Biles II** on the floor.

'Noteworthy'

Record-Breaking: Biles broke records for successive all-around titles as her sustained performance showed that she could compete at the top level over a number of years.

Legacy of Innovation: Her routines and skills helped shape new gymnastics skills as her performances kept pushing the sport's limits.

Rio Olympics 2016

Highlights of Performance- Team Gold: Biles demonstrated her abilities in the team competition, which played a major role in the U.S. team's gold medal victory.

All-Around Gold: With a dominant performance showcasing her technical skill and consistency, she took home the gold medal in the all-around competition.

Mary A.Clapp

Vault Gold: She demonstrated her dominance in this event with her performance on the vault, which included the 'Biles'.

Floor Exercise Gold: Bales' floor routine, which included the 'Biles' and 'Biles II, was praised for its skill and difficulty.

Balance Beam Bronze: Her bronze medal in the balance beam showcased her extraordinary abilities, despite it not being her best event.

Noteworthy

Historic Performance: Biles's accomplishments in Rio solidified her place among the best gymnasts of all time, making her the most decorated gymnast at a single Olympic Games.

Impact on the Sport: Her performance inspired upcoming gymnast generations and established new standards for perfection.

Doha, Qatar: 2018 World Championships

Highlights of Performance- All-Around Gold: Biles triumphed in her comeback, taking home the gold medal for all-around performance.

Vault and Floor Gold: She showed off her sustained excellence and inventiveness in her vault and floor exercises.

Noteworthy

Return to Form: After a brief break, Biles demonstrated her perseverance and capacity to continue performing at her best in this competition, signaling her return to her best.

Ongoing impact: Her performance upheld her reputation as a top gymnast and kept her impact in the sport alive.

World Championships in 2019 (Germany, Stuttgart)

Highlights of Performance- All-Around Gold: Biles set a record at the World Championships by winning her sixth all-around gold.

Mary A.Clapp

Vault and Floor Gold: Maintained her dominance in vault and floor exercises by continuing to excel in these events.

Noteworthy

Record-Breaking: Biles broke records in 2019 by becoming the most decorated gymnast in the history of the World Championships, demonstrating her consistent excellence and influence on the sport.

Legacy: Her feats established new benchmarks for upcoming competitors and cemented her reputation as one of the best gymnasts in history. Key performances by Simone Biles have had a huge impact on the gymnastics community, breaking records and affecting the growth of the sport. Her extraordinary talent, creative routines, and unwavering perfection have made her a legendary figure in gymnastics and an inspiration to gymnasts everywhere.

CHAPTER 10: BEYOND GYMNASTICS

The impact of Simone Biles goes far beyond her gymnastics accomplishments. Her influence may be seen in her advocacy work, contributions to many industries, and personal pursuits, all of which highlight her multidimensional role as a public personality and athlete.

Entertainment and Media

Appearances and Television

Reality TV: In 2017, Simone took part in the 24th season of "Dancing with the Stars," where she attracted new fans and demonstrated her versatility. Her on-show performances demonstrated her versatility and grace outside of gymnastics.

Guest Appearances: Biles has shared her experiences and insights on talk shows, such as "The Ellen DeGeneres Show" and "The Tonight Show Starring Jimmy Fallon."

Media Projects and Documentaries

Documentary Films: "The Simone Biles Story: Courage to Soar," a comprehensive look at Simone's life and accomplishments, is one of the documentaries that highlights Simone's life and career.

Books: She has written a number of books, including the autobiography "Courage to Soar," which describes her experiences and highlights her triumphs.

Activism and Advocacy

Awareness of Mental Health - Open Discussions: Simone has been a strong supporter of mental health, speaking candidly about her personal difficulties and enticing others to get support. Her openness has helped to lessen the stigma associated with mental health problems. Support efforts: She has used her platform to raise awareness and provide resources for mental health issues, supporting organizations and efforts in this area.

Survivor Support

Advocacy for Abuse Survivors: Simone has been a vocal supporter of abuse survivors, especially in the wake of the Larry Nassar crisis. She has advocated for more responsibility and changes both inside and outside the gymnastics community.

Legislative Advocacy: Biles has backed legislative initiatives aimed at enhancing athlete safeguards and boosting openness in athletic associations.

Charity and Involvement in the Community

Volunteering - Foundations and Donations: Simone has supported groups that prioritize health, education, and children, among other charity endeavors. She participates in fundraising activities and makes gifts to charities.

Mary A.Clapp

Community Engagement: She has taken an active part in the community, especially by organizing events and outreach initiatives that serve to uplift and assist youth.

Role modeling and mentoring

Young Athletes: Simone has acted as a mentor to young gymnasts and athletes, offering advice and sharing her experiences to assist them in reaching their objectives. She also coaches others by promoting tenacity and commitment.

Educational Outreach: She has taken part in campaigns and programs aimed at educating the public, emphasizing the value of education, and providing a model for pupils.

Private Life and Hobbies

Credit and Accomplishments- Educational Pursuits: Simone has balanced her athletic career with academic interests and aspirations by pursuing education and personal growth outside of gymnastics.

Mary A.Clapp

Personal Interests: She has mentioned that she enjoys fashion, traveling, and being healthy, among other pastimes and pursuits outside of gymnastics.

Public Persona

Social Media Presence: Simone Biles is active on social media, sharing details about her life, career, and volunteer work. She uses her social media accounts to interact with followers and spread the word about worthy causes.

Public Speaking: Biles has given speeches in front of groups of people about a variety of subjects, including her career as a gymnast and growing past obstacles. The influence of Simone Biles goes well beyond her gymnastics accomplishments.

Her varied talents and dedication to creating a positive impact are demonstrated by her contributions to the media, activism, philanthropy, and personal development. Biles reinforces her legacy as a prominent public figure and role model by inspiring and bringing about change through her efforts and influence.

The role mental health plays in Simone Biles's career and personal life has been significantly impacted by her mental health, which has an impact on both her public activism and performance. The significance of mental health in elite sports and other domains has been underscored by Biles' experiences.

Individual Journeys with Mental Health

Difficulties and Obstacles 'strain and Expectations': Biles's mental health has suffered greatly as a result of the tremendous strain and lofty expectations that are placed on her as a professional gymnast. Stress and anxiety have been exacerbated by the pressure to continue performing at your best as well as the attention of the public and media.

Public Disclosures: Simone Biles has been transparent about her battles with mental health, including pressure from her gymnastics profession and feelings of anxiety. Her candor has brought attention to the difficulties sportsmen confront with their mental health.

Distant from Rivals- Tokyo 2020 Olympics: In order to concentrate on her mental health, Biles decided to withdraw from multiple competitions during the 2020 Tokyo Olympics. This decision was crucial because it demonstrated how important it is to put mental health above competitive achievement.

Self-Care and Recovery: A critical first step in Biles' healing was her resolve to put her mental health first. She showed the value of self-care in high-stress situations by taking time out to tend to her needs and restore her mental fortitude.

Public Impact and Advocacy

Awareness-Building 'Mental Health Advocacy': Simone Biles is now a well-known proponent of raising awareness of mental health issues. She has helped to lessen the stigma associated with mental health concerns, especially in the context of professional sports, by openly sharing her struggles.

Inspiring Others: Biles' candor about her struggles with mental health has encouraged a lot of people to talk about their issues and get support. Her example inspires everyone, especially athletes, to put their mental health first and get help when they need it.

 Backing for Initiatives in Mental Health- Campaigns and Collaborations: Biles has contributed to a number of initiatives and campaigns pertaining to mental health. Her involvement includes campaigning for better mental health services and support systems, working with mental health groups, and taking part in awareness campaigns.

Educational Efforts: She has shared her knowledge and encouraged discussions about the significance of mental health by using her platform to educate others. Her efforts are intended to create an atmosphere that is more sympathetic and supportive of people who are struggling with mental health issues.

Sports and Other Aspects Affected

 Transforming the Discussion 'Athlete Well-Being: Biles' focus on mental health has influenced a wider discussion about athletes' wellbeing. Her acts have prompted coaches and sports organizations to take athletes' mental health more seriously and to provide supportive measures.

Mary A.Clapp

Policy and Practice: Sports organizations are paying more attention to mental health policies as a result of Biles' and other athletes' media exposure. This entails promoting improved mental health services, support networks, and an athlete-centered treatment philosophy that is more empathetic.

Change in Culture 'Breaking Taboos: Simone Biles has contributed to shattering stigmas and promoting a more accepting and encouraging attitude surrounding mental health in sports and society by being transparent about her mental health. Her impact has inspired others to put their mental health first and ask for assistance without worrying about being judged.

Simone Biles's contribution to raising awareness of mental health issues has had a significant effect on society at large as well as the sports industry. Her advocacy work and personal experiences have helped raise awareness of mental health concerns and the importance of providing supportive services.

By putting her own mental health first and speaking out for others, Biles has been a major contributor to the

Mary A.Clapp

development of a more understanding and knowledgeable attitude toward mental health.

SIMONE'S CAMPAIGNS FOR MENTAL HEALTH EXAMINATION

Using her position to confront and de-stigmatize mental health concerns, particularly in the context of sports, Simone Biles has become a potent advocate for mental health awareness. Her public remarks, life experiences, and participation in several programs that promote mental health serve as a hallmark of her advocacy.

Individual Experiences and Professions 'Open Discussions'

'Tokyo 2020 Olympics': Biles made a historic move when she decided to put her mental health first by pulling out of multiple Olympic events. She explained her motivations in public, highlighting the significance of self-care and mental health. Her decision generated a lot of conversation about the demands placed on athletes and the importance of mental health care.

Mary A.Clapp

Social Media and Interviews: Biles has talked about her struggles with anxiety and pressure, as well as other mental health issues, on social media and in interviews. Her candor has prompted others to seek assistance and helped normalize discussions about mental health.

Psychological Function Model—Breaking the Stigma: Biles has been instrumental in eradicating the stigma associated with mental health concerns by being transparent about her struggles. Her prominence as a world-class athlete tackling these issues has had a profound effect on public opinion and comprehension.

Assistance with Mental Health Programs

Partnerships and Initiatives: Biles has teamed with a number of mental health-related organizations and campaigns. Her involvement includes advocating for improved support systems, providing resources, and supporting campaigns that raise awareness of mental health issues. Campaign Participation: She has taken part in awareness-building and conversation-starting campaigns related to mental health. Her backing contributes to the growing awareness of the importance of mental health for general wellbeing.

Instructional Activities 'Advocacy for Resources': Biles has pushed for easier access to support services and resources for mental health. She underlines how important it is for educational institutions and sports leagues to have all-encompassing mental health initiatives.

Public Speaking: Biles shares her experiences and views with audiences while educating them about mental health concerns through speeches and public appearances. Her initiatives are intended to create a more knowledgeable and encouraging atmosphere for people coping with mental health issues.

Effects on Society and Sports

Impact on Culture of Sports - Changing Perceptions: The sports community's perception of mental health has changed as a result of Biles' activism. Discussions regarding the need for an approach to athlete care that is more sympathetic and encouraging have been sparked by her acts.

Policy Changes: Biles's advocacy and the heightened awareness of mental health have contributed to a greater emphasis on mental health policies within sports organizations. This includes enhanced resources and support networks for athletes.

Greater Impact on Society 'Encouraging Dialogue: Biles's initiatives have sparked a more general conversation on mental health in society. Her readiness to discuss these matters in public has aided in the development of a more accepting and candid society surrounding mental health.

Inspiration for Others: Her advocacy has motivated those outside of the athletics world to talk about and get help for mental health issues. Others have been inspired to prioritize mental health by Biles' example, which highlights its significance. The sports industry as well as society at large have been greatly impacted by Simone Biles's activism for mental health awareness.

By breaking the stigma and promoting a more supportive and open conversation about mental health, she has done so through her personal experiences, public declarations, and support for mental health projects. The way that mental health is seen and dealt

Mary A.Clapp

with in a variety of contexts has changed for the better because of Biles' work.

THE IMPACT OF THE "TWISTIES"

The syndrome known as "twisties" affects gymnasts and sportsmen, causing them to lose control and spatial awareness when doing twisting techniques. Both safety and performance may be greatly impacted by this problem. During the 2020 Tokyo Olympics, Simone Biles raised awareness of this problem and demonstrated its significance in the sports world. Recognizing the Contradictions

Explanation and Significance- Spatial Disorientation: Athletes who perform twisties experience a loss of awareness of their body's orientation and position in the air. This may cause confusion and make it harder to carry out challenging actions securely.

Fear and Anxiety: Twister athletes frequently have increased fear and anxiety, which can aggravate the problem and make even simple tasks difficult.

Mary A.Clapp

Performance Impact-Skill Execution: Athletes may find it challenging to accurately execute complex routines due to a loss of spatial awareness. Errors, a drop in performance quality, and a higher chance of injury might arise from this.

Confidence: Athletes who suffer from twisties may feel less confident, which could affect how they perform overall and approach competition.

The Twisties and Simone Biles

2020 Tokyo Olympics - Public Disclosure: Simone Biles talked candidly about her encounter with the twisties at the Tokyo 2020 Olympics. She cited the twisties as a major influence in her choice to prioritize her physical and mental wellbeing, leading her to choose to withdraw from multiple events.

Impact on Performance: Biles's performance at the Olympics was impacted by her battle with the twisties. Her decision to withdraw from competitions brought attention to the difficulties and dangers posed by this illness, highlighting how crucial mental and physical health are to gymnastics.

Mary A.Clapp

 Awareness and Advocacy—Breaking the Silence**:
Biles contributed to increasing awareness of the illness
and its effects on athletes by speaking out about the
twisties. Her candor aided in expanding awareness of
the psychological and physical difficulties gymnasts
confront.

Encouraging Support: Biles's experience brought to light
the necessity for improved support networks for athletes
going through comparable struggles. Discussions
concerning the significance of mental health and safety
in sports have been sparked by her activism.

Effect on the Community of Gymnasts

 Awareness Raised Educational Efforts: The gymnastics
community now knows more about the issue as a result
of Biles' experience with the twisties. The signs and
possible effects of the twisties are now better
understood by coaches, athletes, and sports experts.

Support Systems: The twisties' media attention has
raised attention to the need for better resources and
support systems for athletes going through comparable

struggles. Support for mental health issues and methods for handling spatial disorientation are included in this.

Change in Culture Prioritizing Mental Health: The way mental health and athlete well-being are viewed has changed in part due to Biles' candor with the twisties. Her experience has shown how crucial it is to approach problems with both physical and mental health with compassion and understanding.

Changing Norms: The discourse around the twisties has prompted a reassessment of performance standards and an appreciation of the critical roles that both physical and mental well-being play in sports achievement. Simone Biles's experience with the twisties has raised a lot of awareness about the relationship between mental and physical health in athletics.

The difficulties posed by this illness have been brought to attention by Biles's public disclosure and campaigning, which has also advanced knowledge of how it affects athletes. Her story has led to a transformation in culture that prioritizes mental health and safety in gymnastics and beyond, as well as greater awareness and support.

CHAPTER 11 : LIFE OFF THE MAT

Outside of the gymnastics mat, Simone Biles has a wide variety of interests, pursuits, and contributions that are indicative of her complex character and moral principles. In addition to her gymnastics accomplishments, Biles is well-known for her involvement in a variety of activities and her influence on a range of spheres of life.

Private Life

Relationships and Family- Family Support: Simone Biles has frequently expressed gratitude to her family for providing her with consistent support during her gymnastics career. Her success and well-being have been largely attributed to her ties with her family.

Public connections: Biles has periodically posted peeks of her life with her partner and family on social media and has been upfront about her personal connections.

 Credentials and Hobbies Educational Pursuits: Biles has demonstrated a dedication to learning and self-improvement in spite of her rigorous gymnastics regimen. She has managed to juggle her interests and academic aspirations with her sports career.

Hobbies & Interests: Biles enjoys a variety of things outside of gymnastics, such as fitness, fashion, and travel. She has a strong interest in leading a healthy lifestyle and enjoys traveling to new areas.

Entertainment and Media

 Public Appearances and Television Reality TV: In 2017, Biles took part in the 24th season of the television program "Dancing with the Stars." Her versatility was demonstrated by her performance on the show, which won her admirers outside of the gymnastics community.

Mary A.Clapp

Talk programs and interviews: She has participated in a number of talk programs and interviews, giving insights into her professional background, personal life, and advocacy work.

 Literature and Films- Autobiography: Biles is a writer of books, including "Courage to Soar," her autobiography that offers a detailed look at her life, struggles, and victories.

Documentaries: A thorough look at her life and accomplishments can be found in documentaries like "The Simone Biles Story: Courage to Soar," which highlights her career and life.

Social Action and Charity

 Advocacy for Mental Health-Public Speaking: Biles has advocated for improved support networks for individuals and athletes by using her platform to raise awareness of mental health issues and stress their significance. Campaigns and Collaborations: She has participated in campaigns and initiatives aimed at raising awareness of mental health issues, which has helped to advance knowledge of mental health.

Mary A.Clapp

Volunteering—Foundations and Donations: Biles has contributed to a number of nonprofits, namely those that serve underprivileged youth, the arts, and healthcare. Her involvement in fundraising events and donations are examples of her contributions.

Community Engagement: In an effort to uplift and assist youth, she actively works with communities through outreach initiatives and events.

Public Personas and Social Media

Installation on Social Media Interaction with Followers: Biles is active on social media, sharing information about her life, work, and hobbies. She establishes a connection and provides insight into her personal life through her conversations with followers.

Advocacy and Awareness: She utilizes her social media channels to spread the word about worthwhile causes, such as community service projects and mental health.

Public Image

Role Model: Because of her accomplishments, activism, and uplifting impact, Biles is regarded as a role model. Her public character is a reflection of her perseverance, determination, and devotion to changing many facets of life. Outside of the gymnastics ring, Simone Biles is a vibrant, versatile person who thrives in both the public and private spheres.

Her varied interests and dedication to creating a positive influence are demonstrated by her involvement in activism, charities, and the media. Beyond her sporting accomplishments, Biles' legacy reaches out to inspire and impact others through her personal endeavors and public activities.

Private and public spheres Both Simone Biles' private and public lives exhibit a compelling combination of charm, tenacity, and sincerity. Her impact and legacy have been greatly influenced by her life outside of the gym and the way she portrays herself to the world.

Private Life

History with Family

Adoptive Family: Ron and Nellie Biles, Biles' adoptive grandparents, have been a vital source of support for her throughout her life and professional career. Her family's bond with her has given her stability and strength.

Family Dynamics: Biles frequently talks about her strong relationship with her family, which includes her brothers, and gives them credit for their steadfast encouragement and support.

Credentials and Hobbies - Academic Pursuits: Biles has attempted to further her studies in spite of her demanding gymnastics schedule. Her commitment to academic pursuits and athletics has been well-balanced, demonstrating her commitment to personal development.

Hobbies: Aside from gymnastics, Biles' interests include traveling, being active, and fashion. She is quite interested in traveling to different locations and leading a healthy lifestyle.

Public Image

Involvement and Social Media-Active Presence: Biles shares updates about her life, career, and personal interests on social media channels. Fans can get an insight into her experiences and daily life through her posts.

Connection with Fans: Biles interacts with her fans on social media by offering advice, acknowledging achievements, and bringing up significant topics. She establishes a solid rapport with her audience through her conversations.

Media and Public Appearances Television Appearances: Biles has made appearances on a number of talk shows and reality TV programs. Her performances highlight her adaptability and capacity to engage audiences outside of the gymnastics community.

Interviews and Public Speaking: She has discussed her profession, life experiences, and advocacy work in a number of interviews and public speaking engagements. Her self-assurance and eloquent personality come through in her public speeches.

Influence and Function Model Inspiration: Because of her accomplishments, tenacity, and advocacy, Biles is seen as a role model by many. Many people find inspiration in her tale of overcoming obstacles and excelling at the highest levels of gymnastics.

Advocacy and Awareness: She places a lot of emphasis on advocacy in her public persona, especially in relation to mental health and survivor assistance. Biles is dedicated to changing the world, and she uses her position to spread awareness and encourage good change.

 Self-Portrayal and Personalization—Fashion & Style: Biles has dabbled in a number of fashion-related endeavors and has a noticeable sense of style. Her interest in fashion and personal branding is evident in her public appearances and endorsements.

Brand Collaborations: She has collaborated with businesses and brands, using her public image to support goods and causes that she supports. These partnerships demonstrate her attractiveness and influence outside of gymnastics. Both her private and public personas showcase a sophisticated, multidimensional person who thrives as a public figure and an athlete.

Mary A.Clapp

This is Simone Biles. Her reputation as a personable and inspirational role model is bolstered by her personal interests, tight family ties, and active fan involvement. Through her advocacy work, public appearances, and social media presence, Biles keeps making a big difference and spreading her influence outside of the gymnastics community.

PHILANTHROPY AND INVOLVEMENT WITH THE COMMUNITY

Simone Biles's community service and philanthropic endeavors demonstrate her unwavering commitment to leaving a positive legacy beyond her gymnastics career. Her attempts to interact with communities and support a range of causes are a reflection of her ideals and desire to give back.

Donations to Charities

Academies and Establishments - Simone Biles Foundation: The Simone Biles Foundation works to uplift marginalized communities, families, and children.

Mary A.Clapp

The organization helps young people better their lives and reach their goals by offering resources, support, and scholarships.

Partnerships with Charities: Biles works with a number of nonprofit groups to promote issues including youth development, health, and education. Her alliances frequently involve advocacy, donations, and fundraising occasions.

 Mental Health Support- Mental Health Initiatives: Biles has taken a leading role in promoting resources and awareness for mental health. She collaborates with mental health-focused groups and makes use of her platform to advance awareness of and provide assistance for mental health.

Public Advocacy: Biles has contributed to stigma reduction and awareness-raising by being candid about her personal battles with mental health. She engages in campaigns and events that emphasize the value of mental health as part of her advocacy.

Involvement with the Community

Instructional Engagement- School Visits and Programs: In order to uplift and encourage youngsters, Biles participates in educational programs and school visits. She takes part in activities, delivers talks, and opens up about her experiences to inspire young people to follow their goals and overcome obstacles.

Mentorship: Biles provides advice and support to young athletes and students through a variety of programs. Her mentoring approach is centered on assisting people in realizing their own potential and choosing their own routes to success.

Family and Youth Assistance-Outreach Programs: Biles backs community outreach initiatives that offer kids and families support and services. With the goal of enhancing quality of life, these programs frequently incorporate exercises, seminars, and support services. Community Events: She takes part in fundraising events and other community-related activities, such as charity races. Her participation encourages support and increases exposure for worthy causes.

Public Involvement and Advocacy

Mary A.Clapp

 Assisting Victims of Abuse- Awareness Campaigns: In the wake of the Larry Nassar crisis, Biles has been an outspoken supporter of abuse survivors. She is in favor of programs and campaigns that work to strengthen athlete protections and hold abusers accountable.

Legislative Efforts: As part of her advocacy, she backs legislation aimed at improving athlete safety and openness in sports leagues.

 Encouraging Good Change-Community Impact: Biles' charitable giving and volunteer efforts have a real positive influence on people's lives both locally and globally. Her work addresses a range of societal challenges and promotes progress.

Inspirational Role: Biles is a prominent person who inspires people to perform community service and philanthropy by leveraging her influence. The philanthropy and community service of Simone Biles demonstrate her dedication to changing the world for the better.

 Through her foundation, mental health support, educational outreach, and advocacy work, Biles shows

Mary A.Clapp

that she is committed to uplifting people's lives and tackling significant social concerns. Her ideals and desire to have a positive impact on her community and beyond are reflected in her contributions, which go beyond gymnastics.

CHAPTER 12: CHALLENGES AND TRIUMPHS

Gymnast Simone Biles has faced several notable obstacles along the way, but she has also achieved incredible success. Her career is a testament to her tenacity, willpower, and capacity to overcome setbacks in order to attain extraordinary achievement.

Difficulties

Primary Years and Individual Challenges- Adoptive Background: After being adopted, Biles had to adjust to a new family dynamic. In her early years, she had to overcome obstacles in her family and personal life, including the fallout from her biological mother's hardships.

Balancing Gymnastics and Personal Life: Maintaining balance can be extremely difficult due to the demands of competitive gymnastics, which frequently require balancing rigorous training schedules with obligations to family, friends, and school.

Health Concerns, Mental and Physical Injuries and Physical Strains: Biles has experienced physical strains and injuries throughout her career, just like many other elite athletes. The physical toll of intense training and competition has necessitated cautious recuperation and treatment.

Mental Health Struggles: Biles has been transparent about her battles with anxiety and the twisties, a disorder that throws off her sense of direction when performing twisting moves. Her performance has been affected by these difficulties, and she has had to put her mental health first.

Public Expectations and Pressure- High Expectations: Biles was under tremendous pressure to constantly perform at the best levels because she was a top gymnast. The strain of continuing to perform at a high level was increased by the demands made by sponsors, media, and fans.

Media Scrutiny: Athletes may find it too much to handle the ongoing public attention and media scrutiny. Biles has had to balance the demands of her personal and professional life with the difficulties of being in the public eye.

Victories

Achievements in Gymnastics- Olympic Success: Biles has won four gold medals at the Rio Olympics in 2016 and one bronze medal in Tokyo 2020, demonstrating her incredible success in the games. She became known as one of the finest gymnasts of all time thanks to her performances.

World Championships: Biles has performed admirably in the World Championships, setting records and taking home multiple medals. She has received a great deal of praise for her creative routines and superb technique.

Mary A.Clapp

 Tradition and Innovation-Redefining Gymnastics: The standards of gymnastics have been redefined by Biles' presentation of new and challenging skills. Her inventive routines and distinct abilities have impacted the development of the sport and set new standards.

Enduring Influence: Beyond her accomplishments, Biles has inspired upcoming generations of athletes with her influence on gymnastics. Her achievements in the sport and her standing as an inspiration for tenacity and brilliance will live on in her legacy.

 Action and Significance-Mental Health Awareness: By candidly sharing her experiences and pushing for stronger support networks, Biles has made a major impact on raising awareness of mental health issues. Her bravery in speaking out about mental health has changed people's opinions and created a more encouraging atmosphere.

Philanthropy and Community Involvement: Biles' charitable endeavors and involvement in the community demonstrate her dedication to having a good influence. Her commitment to giving back and championing worthy causes is evident in her work with charities, educational initiatives, and advocacy campaigns.

The journey of Simone Biles is marked by a number of noteworthy setbacks and incredible victories. Her tenacity and determination are demonstrated by her capacity to triumph over social, physical, and personal obstacles while still attaining extraordinary success in gymnastics. Biles has established a lasting legacy through her accomplishments, activism, and charitable endeavors, encouraging others to take on their own obstacles head-on and persevere through them.

2020 Tokyo Olympics For Simone Biles, the 2020 Tokyo Olympics—which were actually held in 2021 because of the COVID-19 pandemic—were a momentous occasion. Her memorable performances, difficulties, and influence on the international scene defined the Games.

Get Ready and Set Your Expectations

Readiness and Training- Intensive Preparation: Biles trained extremely hard in the run-up to the Olympics in Tokyo. She had to undergo rigorous training, physical

Mary A.Clapp

conditioning, and mental toughness in order to be ready to compete at the top level.

Great Expectations: Fans, the media, and the gymnastics community had great expectations for Biles coming into Tokyo as the defending Olympic champion from the 2016 Rio Games. It was expected that she would be a strong candidate to win gold in several different events.

 USA Team and Objectives- Team Dynamics: Along with other exceptional gymnasts, Biles was a vital component of the U.S. gymnastics team. The group wanted to improve on their prior victories and take first place in the competition. Personal Objectives: Biles wanted to retain her titles and possibly increase the number of Olympic medals she already possessed. Her objectives were to do well in individual competitions and add to the team's overall accomplishments.

Difficulties and Retractions

The Twisties and Mental Health Twisties: Biles suffered from a condition known as the twisties during the Games that prevented him from seeing his surroundings when twisting. Her performance suffered as a result, and serious worries about her safety were raised.

Withdrawal from Events: Biles had to make the tough choice to pull out of multiple competitions, including the team final and multiple individual contests, due to the twisties and associated mental health issues. Her choice brought attention to how crucial self-care and mental wellness are in competitive athletics.

Mass Media and Public Responses-Media Coverage: Biles's public disclosure of her difficulties with mental health and her withdrawals were widely covered by the media. Responses varied from encouraging to critical, illustrating the nuanced dynamics of the public scrutiny that prominent athletes must deal with.

Support and Criticism: The public and media had differing opinions about Biles' decision to prioritize her mental health, despite the fact that many people applauded her. The talk emphasized the larger discussion around the demands and expectations made of athletes.

Accomplishments and Displays

Mary A.Clapp

Mullets and Competitions - Balance Beam: Despite her difficulties, Biles participated in the final and took home a bronze medal. Her ability to perform under duress and her perseverance made her performance noteworthy.

Team Event: The United States squad won a silver medal despite Biles being absent from the last rotation. Although Biles made a substantial contribution to the team's previous rounds, her withdrawal had an impact on the outcome.

Effect and Heritage-Raising Awareness: Biles' Olympic experience in Tokyo significantly increased public awareness of mental health concerns in sports. Her candor and choice to put her health first aided in the expansion of the dialogue around the significance of mental health.

Inspiration and Courage: Biles' involvement and advocacy throughout the Games inspired many, despite the difficulties she encountered. Her bravery in talking about mental health and her perseverance in competing in spite of adversity had a profound effect on the public and the sport.

Mary A.Clapp

A pivotal period in Simone Biles' career, the 2020 Tokyo Olympics brought with them both great successes and noteworthy setbacks. Her experience brought to light the difficulties associated with competing at the highest level, as well as the value of mental health and the demands placed on athletes. Biles's support of mental health and her enduring impact on gymnastics and other sports are among her legacies from the Tokyo Games.

OVERCOMING HARDSHOT AND DIFFICULTIES

There have been many difficulties and hardships in Simone Biles' gymnastics career. Her perseverance, tenacity, and strength as an athlete and a person have been demonstrated by her capacity to overcome these challenges.

Individual Challenges

Family and Early Life Challenges - Adoptive Background: Because of her original mother's issues with substance misuse, Biles was adopted by her grandparents, Ron and Nellie Biles. The first hurdles were adjusting to a new family and getting over the effects of her early life.

Financial Struggles: Biles had financial challenges as a child, which would have limited her access to resources and training. Her family's encouragement and tenacity, though, enabled her to carry on with her gymnastics career.

 Combining Requirements—Academic and Athletic Demands: It was difficult to juggle a rigorous gymnastics routine with obligations to my social life and my studies. Biles demonstrated her commitment and time management abilities by succeeding in both areas.

Physical Difficulties

 Physical strain and injuries Injuries: Throughout her career, Biles has had a number of injuries, including back and ankle problems. Careful monitoring, rehabilitation, and modifications to her training program were necessary for every injury.

Mary A.Clapp

Physical Toll: Her body suffered a great deal as a result of the demanding training schedule and competitive demands of professional gymnastics. Sustaining maximum performance under this physical pressure was a constant challenge.

Twisties—Loss of Spatial Awareness: Biles had the twisties at the 2020 Tokyo Olympics, which is a disorder that throws you off when you're twisting. Her participation in events had to be reevaluated due to the hazards this condition posed to both her performance and safety.

Difficulties with Mental Health

Public Expectations and Pressure High Expectations: Biles was under tremendous pressure to continually perform at the best level because she was a star athlete. The mental strain was exacerbated by the weight of expectations from sponsors, media, and supporters.

Media Scrutiny: She may feel overburdened by the media's unceasing focus on her performances and private life. Under such circumstances, preserving mental health and controlling public perception presented formidable obstacles.

 Advocacy for Mental Health Personal Struggles: Biles has been candid about her battles with mental illness and anxiety, especially in stressful circumstances. Her readiness to speak out about these concerns in public has served as a platform for advocacy as well as a personal hardship.

Advocacy Efforts: Biles has influenced a wider discussion on the significance of mental well-being in sports and other domains by emphasizing her mental health and pushing for mental health awareness.

Victories and Fortitude

 Success Despite Difficulties Olympic Success: Biles has had incredible success, including many Olympic gold medals and world championships, in spite of adversity. Her ability to bounce back from setbacks has been a key component of her success.

Innovation and Excellence: Biles has redefined the norms of gymnastics by introducing new skills and methods. Her extraordinary intellect and tenacity are highlighted by her capacity for innovation and success in the face of adversity.

Impact and Inspiration- Role Model: Biles is a role model for many people because of her capacity to overcome obstacles on the personal, physical, and mental levels. Her story exemplifies the value of resilience, willpower, and self-care.

Advocacy and Influence: Biles has utilized her platform to improve the lives of others by supporting mental health and philanthropy. Her bravery in facing and conquering hardship has motivated a lot of people to take on their own obstacles. The story of Simone Biles is a potent example of overcoming hardship and obstacles.

Her capacity to overcome obstacles—mental, physical, and personal—while attaining extraordinary achievement demonstrates her fortitude and tenacity. Through her experiences, Biles not only draws attention to her own accomplishments but also advances crucial discussions about mental health and the wider effects of overcoming adversity.

Mary A.Clapp

HARMONIZING INDIVIDUAL AND WORK-RELATED PRESSURES

Throughout her gymnastics career, Simone Biles has had to reconcile her demanding work schedule with a healthy personal life. Her success and well-being have greatly depended on her capacity to handle these stresses.

Pressures in the Workplace

Excellent Performance and Expectations-Elite Competition: Being one of the best gymnasts in the world, Biles has tremendous pressure to continually deliver her best work. A constant in her career is the pressure to continue performing at her best on both a physical and mental level.

Media Scrutiny: She is under more strain due to the extensive media attention and public interest in her performances. In addition to concentrating on her training and contests, Biles has to control media expectations and public perceptions.

Mary A.Clapp

Injury Management and Training- Difficult Training:
Biles has an intense training schedule that calls for
hours of repetition, conditioning, and skill improvement.
To continue performing at your best, you must strike a
balance between this demanding schedule and
relaxation and recuperation.

Injury Prevention and Recovery: A big part of her work
life is handling physical strain and injuries. Biles has to
manage the difficulties of avoiding injuries, getting well
after her recovery, and keeping up her general physical
condition.

Individual Stressors Social and Family Life - Family
Dynamics: Biles comes from a close-knit family that is
very important to her. It takes meticulous time
management and the support of her loved ones for her
to juggle the demands of her gymnastics career with her
family's obligations and relationships.

Social Life: Because of her hectic schedule, she may
find it difficult to maintain a social life and pursue
hobbies outside of gymnastics. Biles needs to figure out
how to strike a balance between her social life and her
work obligations.

Mary A.Clapp

Psychological Health and Welfare-Mental Health Management: Public scrutiny and the demands of top competition can have an adverse effect on mental health. Biles has been transparent about her battles with anxiety and the significance of putting her mental health and well-being before her work obligations.

Self-Care: Stress management and self-care are essential to juggling the demands of both personal and professional life. Biles uses coping mechanisms to keep her mental and emotional well-being in check, such as asking for help and making time for herself.

Techniques for Maintaining Balance

Organization of Time - organized Schedule: Biles manages her training, competitions, and personal life with an organized schedule. She can better manage her time and balance the demands of her personal and professional obligations.

Prioritization: Managing demands from the workplace and personal spheres requires prioritizing tasks and establishing boundaries. In order to achieve her goals and maintain balance, Biles concentrates on important aspects of her life and career.

Support Systems

Family Support: Biles's family offers stability and encouragement, which is a vital source of support. Their participation aids in her ability to balance her personal and professional obligations. Professional Support: Biles overcomes the difficulties of elite competition by collaborating with trainers, coaches, and mental health specialists. Their assistance is essential for handling the demands of performance and preserving general wellbeing.

Awareness of Mental Health-Open Communication: Biles' candidness regarding her battles with mental health issues helps people recognize the significance of mental health. She lowers stigma and inspires people to put their mental health first by speaking honestly.

Advocacy: Biles's support of mental health awareness campaigns helps her manage the demands of both her personal and professional lives. Her talks in public about mental health add to the larger dialogue about support and self-care.

Simone Biles's perseverance and adept management are demonstrated by her ability to manage the demands of both her personal and professional lives. Through the use of time management techniques, utilizing support networks, and placing mental health first, Biles is able to balance her demanding professional gymnastics schedule with her personal life. Her experiences provide insightful advice on how to balance the demands of elite competition with one's own well-being.

CHAPTER 13: RETURN TO COMPETITION

After going through difficult times and recovering, Simone Biles has shown resiliency, tenacity, and adaptability in her comeback to competition. Her recovery is evidence of her fortitude and commitment to the game.

Recuperation and Readiness

 After the Olympics- Mental Health Focus: Biles purposefully withdrew from competition following the Tokyo 2020 Olympics in order to concentrate on her mental well-being and recuperation. She was able to prioritize her well-being and handle the difficulties she was facing during this time.

Physical Rehabilitation: In order to heal from any injuries and make sure she was physically ready to return to competitive gymnastics, Biles also underwent physical rehabilitation during her absence.

Resuming Training- Gradual Reintegration: Biles eased back into training after opting to compete again. Regaining her competitive edge, strengthening her body, and modifying her routines were all part of this process.

Skill Refinement: Following her break from competitive gymnastics, Biles focused on honing her routines and talents, adding new components, and resolving any necessary technical improvements.

Return of the Competition

Domestic and Global Events- U.S. Gymnastics Championships: Biles returned to the scene at the U.S. Gymnastics Championships, showcasing her abilities and preparedness for competition. Her comeback to peak form was meticulously monitored by watching her performances.

 Foreign competitions: As part of her return, Biles took part in foreign competitions. These contests gave her the chance to demonstrate her abilities on a worldwide scale and determine whether she was ready for more competitive events.

 Highlights of Performance Notable Performances: Biles made a triumphant comeback to competition, showcasing her unwavering greatness and versatility. Her performances demonstrated her technical skill as well as her capacity to execute well under duress.

Medals and Placements: Biles' comeback was characterized by outstanding performances, including high placements and medal finishes. Her performance confirmed her place among the world's best gymnasts.

Difficulties and Modifications

Adapting to Modifications Mental and Physical Adjustments: She had to adapt to changes in both her physical and mental well-being in order to compete again. Biles had to deal with the demands of competitive gymnastics, adjust to new routines, and handle any aftereffects of her sabbatical.

Public Expectations: Biles had a lot of expectations from the public because she is a well-known athlete. It took careful management to strike a balance between her personal aspirations and well-being and their demands.

Continuous Attention to Mental Health-Continued Advocacy: Throughout her recovery, Biles has persisted in promoting self-care and mental health awareness. Her attitude toward competition and preparation continues to be centered around her mental wellness.

Support Systems: Her successful comeback has depended on her ability to keep a solid support network, which includes family, coaches, and mental health specialists. She is able to handle the pressures of competitiveness and personal obstacles thanks to these supports.

Legacy and Significance

Mary A.Clapp

Influence and Motivation-Role Model: Many athletes and others have been motivated by Biles's comeback to competition. Her capacity to bounce back from setbacks and resume her form shows tenacity and resolve.

Impact on Gymnastics: She is still having an impact on the sport of gymnastics, both in terms of performance expectations and the ongoing discussion surrounding mental health and the welfare of athletes.

Goals for the Future- Career Goals: Looking ahead, Biles hopes to continue to succeed in gymnastics, maybe compete in the future, and continue to give back to the community and sport.

Continued Advocacy: Biles intends to use her position to inspire others and bring about positive change in the areas of mental health and support for athletes. Simone Biles's decision to compete again is a testament to her incredible tenacity and commitment. She was able to successfully reintegrate into the competitive gymnastics landscape by addressing both her physical and mental concerns.

Mary A.Clapp

Her return not only demonstrates her inner strength but also solidifies her position as a prominent athlete and mental health advocate.

Retirement in 2023: After taking a break after the Tokyo 2020 Olympics, Simone Biles's comeback in 2023 demonstrated her perseverance and unwavering excellence, marking a pivotal juncture in her gymnastics career.

Getting Ready for the Reentry

Resuming Training concentrated Training: Biles concentrated on improving her competitive edge in the run-up to her 2023 comeback. This involved strengthening her muscles, honing her techniques, and being ready both psychologically and physically for the rigors of elite competition.

Mental Health Considerations: As part of her training, Biles kept her mental health as a top priority. This required collaborating with mental health specialists and using stress management and wellbeing-preserving techniques.

Mary A.Clapp

 Public Declaration—Disclosing Plans: The public and media were eager to learn that Biles would be making a comeback to competitive gymnastics. The gymnastics community, as well as her supporters, greeted her return with enthusiasm and support.

HIGHLIGHTS OF THE COMPETITION

 Championships for US Gymnastics-Performance: Biles displayed her abilities with powerful performances at the 2023 U.S. Gymnastics Championships. Her performances showed off her technical skill and ability to adjust following her break from competition.

Outcomes: Biles turned in a remarkable performance, taking home first place and solidifying her spot among the world's best gymnasts. Her preparation and commitment were evident in her performance.

International Contests

World Championships: Biles participated in international competitions with the goal of leaving a lasting impression, such as the World Championships. Her involvement in these competitions demonstrated her preparedness to compete internationally. Medals and Placements: In international events, Biles produced noteworthy outcomes, including top finishes and medal wins. Her accomplishments demonstrated her ongoing brilliance and impact in the field.

Difficulties and Adjustments

Switching with the Times Routine Modifications: She had to adjust to new routines and technical components in order to compete again. Biles has to modify her performances to account for any advancements or changes in her abilities.

Physical and Mental Adaptation: Biles made an effort to adjust her body and mind to the rigorous requirements of competitive gymnastics. Maintaining both personal wellbeing and competitive performance required managing these changes.

Mass Media and Public Responses-Media Coverage: The media enthusiastically and critically covered Biles's return. The attention she received from the public and media emphasized the importance of her comeback and the influence of her performances.

Support and Criticism: Although many people were happy to have Biles back, she was also scrutinized and held to high standards. It took careful maneuvering to strike a balance between her personal aspirations, struggles, and public impressions.

Legacy and Significance

Influence and Motivation - Role Model: Biles' triumphant return to the sport inspires people and athletes around him. Her ability to bounce back and perform at her best is a testament to her commitment and tenacity.

Impact on Gymnastics: Her return to the sport has not stopped having an impact, raising the bar for performance and influencing continuous conversations about the health and welfare of athletes.

 Goals for the Future Continued Performance: Biles hopes to compete in events down the road and to maintain her current level of gymnastics performance. Her return paves the way for her continued involvement in the sport.

 Advocacy and Community Engagement: Biles is still dedicated to promoting mental health and being involved in the community. She uses her platform to encourage people and promote worthy organizations. The year 2023 saw Simone Biles make a triumphant return to the gymnastics world.

Biles proved her excellence and resilience with her well-planned performances, consistent dedication to her mental health, and resilient preparation. Her comeback served as a testament to her ongoing gymnastics prowess as well as a symbol of her influence in the sport and her support for the welfare of athletes.

Maintaining Push Restrictions Gymnast Simone Biles has continuously pushed the sport's bounds, creating new norms and redefining what is achievable. Her dedication to creativity and quality has had a significant influence on gymnastics and other sports.

Gymnastics Innovations

New Methods and Abilities Introducing New Ability**: Biles has raised the bar for gymnastics difficulty with a number of ground-breaking abilities. The Biles, a double layout with a half-twist, and the Biles II, a triple-twisting double backflip, are two notable instances. These components show that she can push the boundaries of what is technically possible.

Skill Refinement: Biles has continuously improved and honed her routines in addition to learning new ones. Her focus on accuracy and execution has raised the bar for gymnastics performance.

Rewriting the Handbook

Difficulty Ratings: Biles has impacted gymnastics' difficulty ratings and scores by utilizing her special talents. The code of points has been updated as a result of her performances to match the changing standards in the sport.

Improving Performance Criteria: Biles' inventions have motivated other gymnasts to surpass their own limitations. Her efforts have raised gymnastics' overall performance standards and inspired a new generation of competitors to try out novel routines and methods.

Effect on Athletics Creating New Reference Points Competition Results: Biles' accomplishments, including her several titles at the Olympics and World Championships, have raised the bar for gymnastics success. She has established herself as one of the greatest gymnasts of all time with her consistently outstanding performances.

Influence on Training: gymnasts' competition preparation has been impacted by her method of skill development and training. Innovative routines and a high degree of difficulty have been central to training programs worldwide.

Motivating Next Generations-Role Model: Young gymnasts are inspired by Biles' groundbreaking accomplishments. Her accomplishments inspire young athletes to set high goals and challenge themselves, promoting a culture of creativity and quality in the sport.

Mentorship and Support: Biles helps aspiring athletes by serving as a mentor and by advocating for gymnastics through her participation in the sport. Her leadership guarantees that the tradition of pushing limits continues and contributes to the future development of gymnastics.

Surmounting Obstacles and Adjusting

Survival Despite Obstacles - Adapting to Challenges: Biles has faced difficulties throughout her career, including setbacks with her health and injuries. Her tenacity and resolve are evident in her ability to get past these setbacks and keep pushing the envelope.

Adaptation and Evolution: Biles has modified her strategy and persisted in innovating in the face of obstacles. Her determination to push gymnastics' boundaries is evident in her ability to bounce back from setbacks.

MOVING FORWARD WHILE MAINTAINING WELL-BEING

Prioritizing Health: Biles stresses the significance of striking a balance between innovation and one's own health and well-being while pushing the envelope. Her strategy for maintaining long-term success involves controlling both physical and mental demands.

Ongoing Development: Biles's persistent emphasis on her health and performance guarantees that her innovations are long-lasting and that she will be able to make a significant contribution to the sport going forward.

Legacy and Goals for the Future

Persistent Heritage- Historical Impact: Biles has made a significant and enduring impact on gymnastics. Her accomplishments and innovations have revolutionized the sport and established new benchmarks for upcoming generations.

Mary A.Clapp

Influence on Gymnastics Culture: Her influence goes beyond her performances; she has shaped the sport's ethos and created a welcoming atmosphere where pushing limits is embraced.

Future Objectives

Continued Excellence: Biles wants to keep improving her gymnastics skills while pursuing new avenues and raising her bar for performance.

Advocacy and Growth: Biles is dedicated to advocating for the expansion of gymnastics, in addition to her competitive aspirations. Her goals for the future include encouraging people to push their own boundaries and making a positive impact on the sport.

Gymnastics has changed significantly as a result of Simone Biles' dedication to pushing the sport's bounds. By means of her inventive abilities, she has expanded the boundaries of gymnastics and inspired a new generation of athletes. Her legacy of pushing limits will continue to impact and elevate the sport for years to come, thanks to her perseverance, adaptability, and focus on both performance and well-being.

CHAPTER 14: LEGACY AND INFLUENCE

Simone Biles has left a lasting legacy in gymnastics and beyond, thanks to her ground-breaking accomplishments, impact on the sport, and motivational influence on people all over the world. Beyond her achievements in competition, she has made significant contributions to defining gymnastics' future and advancing moral principles.

 Athletic Accomplishments Rewriting Records in Gymnastics - Record-Breaking Performances: Biles has broken multiple records, including the most gold medals won at World Championships and the most medals won overall. Her feats have raised the bar for gymnastics' caliber and difficulty.

Historic Olympic Success: Biles has cemented her status as one of the most successful gymnasts in Olympic history by winning numerous gold medals. Her performances at the Olympics in Rio de Janeiro (2016) and Tokyo 2020 demonstrate her extraordinary talent and supremacy in competition.

 Creative Ability- New Talents and Elements: Biles has expanded the realm of what is technically feasible in gymnastics by introducing new talents like the Biles and Biles II. The scoring and difficulty requirements for the sport have been impacted by these improvements.

Elevating Performance Standards: Her exceptional routines and technical skill have raised the standard for gymnastics performance, encouraging athletes to aim for more challenging and imaginative routines.

Gymnastics' Impact

Impact on Methods and Training Moderating Training Approaches: Due to Biles's success, training approaches have changed, placing a greater emphasis on challenging routines and cutting-edge methods. Her method has affected coaching techniques and training plans all around the world.

Evolution of the Code of Points: As a result of her performances, the gymnastics code of points has been updated to reflect the changing levels of difficulty and execution in the sport.

Models for Upcoming Generations—Role Model for Young Athletes: Biles' accomplishments and tenacity provide a compelling model for aspiring gymnasts. Her narrative inspires young athletes to reach their goals and test their boundaries, promoting a culture of excellence and aspiration.

Mentorship and Support: Biles helps aspiring athletes by mentoring and supporting them through her involvement in gymnastics and public life. Her mentoring aids in the

Mary A.Clapp

development of the next generation of gymnasts and advances the sport.

Social Impact and Advocacy

Encouraging Awareness of Mental Health

Advocacy for Mental Health: Biles has emphasized the value of self-care and support for athletes by using her platform to promote mental health awareness. Her candor regarding her issues with mental health has aided in expanding the dialogue regarding mental health in sports.

Reducing Stigma: By being transparent about her struggles, Biles has aided in lessening the stigma associated with mental illness and inspired others to put their health first.

Community Service and Philanthropy

Community Involvement: Biles takes an active part in charitable endeavors and neighborhood projects. Her donations promote a number of issues, such as youth development, health, and education.

Mary A.Clapp

Creating chances: Biles supports causes that are in line with her experiences and values and works to provide chances for marginalized populations through her philanthropic work.

Sport's Legacy Permanent Influence on Gymnastics Culture

Redefining Success: Biles' accomplishments have changed the definition of success in gymnastics by establishing new benchmarks for difficulty, performance, and creativity.

Legacy of Excellence: Her influence goes beyond her competitive career, impacting gymnastics culture and motivating competing athletes to push limits and strive for excellence in the future.

Goals for the Future and Persistent Impact

Ongoing Contributions: Biles intends to keep up her advocacy work and gymnastics participation, helping to advance the sport and promoting worthy causes. Inspiration and Influence: Her legacy will keep motivating people and athletes by advancing resilience, creativity, and mental health awareness. The outstanding athletic accomplishments, ground-breaking discoveries, and significant impact on gymnastics and society define Simone Biles' legacy.

Her achievements have revolutionized the sport, motivated upcoming generations, and advanced significant ideals like community support and mental health awareness. The long-lasting influence of Simone Biles will continue to influence gymnastics' future and motivate people everywhere. Role Model and Trailblazer Simone Biles is regarded as a trailblazer and a role model who has influenced gymnastics and other fields through her accomplishments, activism, and self-belief. Her influence goes well beyond her achievements in competition; she has inspired people all across the world and shaped the sport's future.

Setting New Records Creative Works Associated with Gymnastics- Pioneering Skills: Biles is credited for creating and perfecting a number of gymnastics firsts, including the Biles and Biles II, which have raised the bar for difficulty and technique and expanded the realm of what is practical in the sport.

Mary A.Clapp

Elevating Performance Standards: Her routines and techniques have inspired gymnasts to try new things and have lifted the bar for gymnastics greatness. The sport's changing standards and expectations are clearly influenced by Biles.

 Difficult Norms—Redefining Difficulty: Biles has changed the way that gymnastics is seen by incorporating intricate and novel components into her routines. Her method has affected scoring schemes and the code of points, which reflects her influence on the development of the sport.

Breaking Records: Her unprecedented accomplishments, which include the greatest number of World Championship titles and Olympic medals, have raised the bar for success. The achievements of gymnast Simone Biles defy preconceived ideas about what is possible in the sport.

 Motivational Mentor Modeling Determination and Resilience—Overcoming Adversity: Biles's tenacity and resolve are evident in her capacity to overcome obstacles in her personal and professional life, including injuries and mental health issues. Her path is a striking illustration of tenacity and fortitude.

Commitment to Excellence: She demonstrates a strong work ethic and a commitment to excellence via her commitment to training and performance. Biles's passion for the sport and her unwavering drive for betterment have contributed to her success.

Empowerment and Advocacy-Mental Health Awareness: One important part of Biles's role as a role model has been her advocacy for mental health. By being transparent about her struggles with mental health, she has increased awareness and inspired others to put their health first.

Empowering Others: Biles' accomplishments and public advocacy enable people to take on obstacles and pursue their own objectives. People are inspired to pursue their goals, be resilient, and look for help by her example. Impact Outside of Gymnastics Community Service and Philanthropy Charitable Work: Biles actively supports a range of issues, including youth development, health, and education. Her philanthropic endeavors serve to improve communities and demonstrate her dedication to changing the world. Mentorship and Support: Biles assists young people and aspiring athletes by way of public appearances and mentoring. Her mentoring supports and nurtures potential, inspiring the upcoming generation of gymnasts and other leaders.

Affect on Society and Culture—Redefining Success: By defying conventional notions of success, Biles' achievements encourage others to strive for excellence in their own domains. She has influenced cultural ideas of success and talent that go beyond gymnastics. Cultural Impact: One aspect of Biles' influence on popular culture is her standing as a public advocate for significant causes. Her appearance in the media and public debate advances larger discussions on resilience, empowerment, and mental health.

 Legacy and Ongoing Impact Persistent Heritage-Legacy of Innovation: Biles' innovations and excellence have left a long-lasting legacy in gymnastics. Future generations of athletes will be shaped by her impact, which will continue to raise the bar for skill and performance. Role Model for Generations: Future generations of athletes and people will be motivated by Biles's example as a trailblazer and role model. Her influence on gymnastics and society highlights her position as a trailblazer in the promotion of excellence, advocacy, and resilient ideals.

Goals for the Future- Ongoing Contributions: Biles is still dedicated to her work in philanthropy, advocacy, and gymnastics. Her goals for the future include carrying on inspiring others and supporting worthy causes. Inspiration and Impact: People will be motivated to pursue their dreams, overcome obstacles, and have a good impact on their communities by her legacy as a trailblazer and role model.

Simone Biles is an inspiration and trailblazer who has had a lasting impact via her advocacy, tenacity, and ground-breaking accomplishments. Her impact goes beyond gymnastics; she inspires people all across the world and shapes the sport's future. Biles' legacy as a trailblazer and leader is a testament to her unwavering pursuit of perfection and her determination to have a positive social influence.

Mary A.Clapp

ENTRAINING THE FUTURE SCIENCE

The impact of Simone Biles goes much beyond her gymnastics accomplishments; she is a major inspiration to the upcoming generation of athletes and people in general. Her experience as an advocate and a champion provides insightful insights and inspiration for young people who want to achieve their dreams.

 Young Athletes' Role Model Modeling Commitment and Vigor- Dedication to Training: Biles' unwavering focus on her performance and training highlights the value of tenacity and hard work. Her meticulous planning and methodical approach demonstrate the work necessary to succeed in any industry.

Setting High Standards: Her accomplishments serve as an example of how hard work, determination, and a willingness to go beyond one's comfort zone are necessary for excellence, and they set a high bar for aspiring athletes.

Mastering Difficulties—Resilience and Perseverance: Biles is a great example of resilience because of her capacity to overcome obstacles in her personal and professional life, including injuries and mental health issues. Her narrative instills in young athletes the virtue of tenacity in the face of difficulty.

Embracing Failure as a Learning Experience: Biles inspires young people to see failure as a stepping stone to success by sharing her personal experiences with setbacks and recovery. Her strategy for conquering setbacks teaches important lessons about growth and perseverance.

Empowerment and Advocacy Encouraging Awareness of Mental Health- Open Dialogue: By being transparent about her struggles with mental health, Biles has normalized discussions about mental health. Her activism inspires youth to put mental health first and get help when they need it. Encouraging Self-Care: She emphasizes the value of mental health and self-care, highlighting the necessity of keeping a balanced perspective on both competition and personal well-being. Young athletes are encouraged by this message to look out for their physical and mental well-being.

Young People Empowered-Belief in Potential**: Young people are inspired to believe in their own potential by Biles' advocacy and accomplishments. Her success story shows that people may reach their goals if they have perseverance, hard work, and self-belief. Encouraging Pursuit of Dreams: Biles inspires young people to follow their passions and establish lofty objectives by sharing her experience. They are inspired to pursue their goals with boldness by her example.

 Neighborhood and Charity Beneficial Effects on Communities-Philanthropic Efforts: Biles emphasizes the value of helping others and giving back through her participation in community service projects and charitable endeavors. Her numerous charitable endeavors serve as an example of the beneficial effects one person may have on their community. Mentorship and Support: Biles offers advice and assistance to aspiring athletes via her public appearances and mentorship. The future of gymnastics and other disciplines is shaped by her ability to identify talent and provide guidance.

Generating Prospects—Supporting Education and Development: Biles frequently addresses youth development and education in his charitable endeavors. Her initiatives give young people access to tools and initiatives that support their development and achievement. Inspiring Social Change: Biles inspires young people to get involved in their communities and have a good impact on society by championing key causes like social justice and mental health.

 Legacy and Prospective Impact Persistent Motivation Lasting Impact: Future generations will continue to be inspired by Biles' legacy of brilliance, tenacity, and advocacy. Beyond her athletic accomplishments, she has a profound impact on the ideals and goals of youth globally. Excellent Example for Excellence: Biles is a shining example of commitment, tenacity, and empathy. Young people who aspire to improve their own lives and communities might learn from her example.

Goals for the Future-Persistent Impact: Biles's continued participation in charity, gymnastics, and activism will motivate and uplift the coming generation. Her future pursuits will add even more to her outstanding reputation and beneficial influence.Encouraging Future Leaders: Biles inspires the next generation of people who want to greatness and make significant contributions to society by modeling leadership and motivating young people to follow in her footsteps.

The impact of Simone Biles on the upcoming generation is significant and wide-ranging. Young athletes and individuals find great inspiration from her activism, perseverance, and determination. Biles promotes the pursuit of goals and the significance of having a good influence by living according to the ideals of diligence, self-care, and perseverance. Future generations will continue to be shaped and inspired by her legacy, which will uphold excellence, a sense of empowerment, and community involvement.

SLIPPERING DEGARS FOR WOMEN IN SPORTS

Mary A.Clapp

As a trailblazer for better gender equality and visibility, Simone Biles has been instrumental in shattering stereotypes and advancing opportunities for women in sports. Her efforts and accomplishments have had a significant influence on how people view and engage with women in sports.

 Defying Gender Conventions Reinventing Athletic Greatness- Exceptional Performance: Biles' extraordinary gymnastics success has reshaped the expectations for what is deemed feasible for female athletes. Her accomplishments dispel outdated ideas about women's potential in athletics and demonstrate that they can compete at the highest levels. Innovative feats: Biles has pushed the limits of gymnastics' difficulty and technique by developing and mastering intricate feats. Her accomplishments demonstrate that women are just as capable of ingenuity and brilliance as men.

Dispelling Preconceptions-Strength and Power: Biles dispels misconceptions about female athletes with her strength and athleticism. Her strength and technical proficiency show that women can be strong and dominate in sports that are typically thought to be less appropriate for female athletes. Overcoming Bias: In gymnastics and in sports in general, Biles has faced and overcome prejudices. Her accomplishments have aided in changing perceptions and raising awareness of the worth and potential of female athletes.

Effect on Parity of Gender -Progressing Inclusion- Visibility and Recognition: Due to Biles's prominence in the sport, female gymnasts and athletes in general are more visible. Her accomplishments have increased awareness of women's sports and helped to improve the representation of female athletes in the public and media. Role Model for Young Women: Biles is a prominent gymnastics star who acts as a role model for young ladies who want to excel in athletics. A new generation of female athletes is motivated by her accomplishments to follow their passions and overcome obstacles.

Shaping Culture Around Sports-Inspiring Change: Biles has a lasting impact on sports culture, changing how people view and respect female athletes through her example. Her efforts and accomplishments support a larger trend in athletics toward gender equality.

Mary A.Clapp

Promoting Opportunities: Her accomplishments and advocacy work to advance improved facilities, more financing, and more support for female athletes, among other things, for women in sports.

Supporting Gender Equality Advocacy for Women's Rights - Voicing Concerns: Biles has raised awareness of systemic problems and gender inequity that impact female athletes by using her platform to voice her concerns. Her advocacy pushes conversations and increases awareness of significant gender-related issues. Supporting Equal Opportunities: Biles backs programs meant to bring about gender balance in athletics through her words and deeds. Her participation in advocacy work supports the continuous movement to give female athletes equal rights and respect.

Encouraging Mental Wellness and Health—Addressing Mental Health: Biles' candidness regarding her battles with mental health has brought attention to how crucial mental health is for female athletes. Her support of mental health is part of a larger effort to address and give priority to mental health in sports, which helps to create a more encouraging atmosphere for all athletes.

 Legacy and Ongoing Impact Persistent Effect - Changing Perceptions: The way that people view and regard women in sports has been significantly influenced by the accomplishments and activism of Alicia Biles. Stereotypes are still being contested by her impact, and gender equality in sports is being promoted. Inspiring Future Generations: Future generations of female athletes can draw inspiration from her legacy. Young women are inspired by Biles to follow their athletic dreams and overcome obstacles, which helps to create a more diverse and equal sports environment.

Goals for the Future- Ongoing Advocacy: Biles is probably going to keep pushing for women's rights in sports and gender equality. Her upcoming initiatives will help achieve gender balance and assist female athletes to a greater extent. Continued Leadership: As a trailblazer and role model, Biles' leadership will propel good change in the sports industry by inspiring and influencing the upcoming generation of athletes and activists.

Simone Biles has significantly contributed to the advancement of gender equality, dispelling myths, and breaking down obstacles for women in sports. Her accomplishments, activism, and leadership have changed how people view female athletes and made the sports world more welcoming and equal. The legacy of Monica Biles will keep pushing for more chances and representation for women in sports.

Mary A.Clapp

CHAPTER 15: THE BILES EFFECT

The term "Biles Effect" describes the significant influence that Simone Biles's remarkable accomplishments, creative innovations, and activism have had on gymnastics and the larger sports community. This phrase perfectly sums up Biles's varied impact, which has changed people's opinions, motivated next-generation athletes, and improved sports culture.

 Redefinishing Gymnastics Performance Innovation - New Skills and Routines: Biles has created and honed a number of ground-breaking skills that have redefined the bar for gymnastics difficulty, including the Biles and Biles

II. Her creative routines have raised the bar for technical performance and changed the way gymnasts prepare for them. Setting New Benchmarks: Her accomplishments, which include many medals from the Olympics and World Championships, have raised the bar for success. The increased expectations and standards in the sport are a direct result of the Biles Effect.

Scoring and Technique Influencing-Revising the Code of Points: Due to Biles's performances, the gymnastics code of points has been updated to reflect the difficulty and intricacy of her routines, which have become more challenging. Her influence has had a direct impact on gymnastics performance evaluation and scoring methods. Encouraging Technical Evolution: By stretching the bounds of what is technically feasible, Biles has encouraged other gymnasts to experiment with and incorporate novel approaches, creating a climate in which the sport is always evolving.

Effect on Female Sportspeople - Shattering Gender Stereotypes-Breaking Stereotypes: Biles has disproved conventional beliefs about female athletes by demonstrating that they are capable of amazing feats of power, skill, and creativity. Her accomplishments support a more accepting image of female athleticism and serve to destroy antiquated stereotypes. Increasing Visibility: Her notoriety has increased the visibility of female athletes and gymnasts, which has helped to increase the general acknowledgement of women's sporting accomplishments.

Promoting Equality-Encouraging Gender Equality: Biles' support of gender parity in athletics has brought attention to persistent problems and sparked conversations about fair treatment and acknowledgement of female athletes. Her initiatives help the larger push for gender equality. Addressing Mental Health: Her candor on mental health issues has shaped how the sports world views athlete well-being and fostered a more accepting and understanding atmosphere.

Inspirational Guidance Young Athletes: A Role Model-Encouraging Aspiration: Young athletes find great motivation in Biles' accomplishments and tenacity. Aspiring gymnasts and athletes are inspired by her example to work hard and persistently towards their goals. Promoting Self-Belief: Biles inspires young people to have faith in their own skills and pursue greatness by showing what is achievable through perseverance and self-belief.

Affect on Culture of Sports - Building a Culture of Excellence: The Biles Effect reaches into the larger sports world, where her resilience, ingenuity, and excellence are encouraged by her example. Her impact inspires athletes in a variety of disciplines to push boundaries and establish new benchmarks. Advancing Social Change: By influencing the conversation on athlete representation and well-being, Biles' support of gender equality and mental health advances positive social change.

 Legacy and Prospective Impact - Persistent Effect—Shaping the Future of Gymnastics: The Biles Effect will keep influencing gymnastics going forward by motivating upcoming generations of athletes to try out novel tactics and pursue perfection. The changing rules and procedures in the sport are a testament to her legacy. Continued Advocacy: Biles' persistent support of significant causes, such as gender equality and mental health, is expected to have a positive impact on these fields and propel advancements, fostering an atmosphere in athletics that is more welcoming and encouraging.

Motivating Next Generations-Legacy of Inspiration: For upcoming generations of athletes and people, the Biles Effect is an enduring source of motivation. Her activism and accomplishments show that it is possible to soar to new heights and make significant contributions to both sports and society. The revolutionary influence of Simone Biles on gymnastics and sports culture is referred to as the Biles Effect.

Through her advocacy, ingenuity, and outstanding accomplishments, Biles has broken down barriers, disproved myths, and motivated a great number of people. Her impact is felt outside of the sport as well, propelling advancement and cultivating an inclusive and high-achieving culture. The Biles Effect will keep influencing gymnastics' future and motivating upcoming generations of competitors and supporters.

Mary A.Clapp

HOW SIMONE PERMANENTLY CHANGED THE GYM

Simone Biles's tremendous talent, creative talents, and activism have had an unequalled impact on gymnastics, altering the sport in several important ways. Beyond her achievements in competition, she has had a transformative impact on gymnastics off the mat as well.

Trailblazing Concepts New Skill Introduction Groundbreaking Elements: Biles has raised the technical difficulty of routines by introducing a number of new abilities, including the Biles (a double layout with a half twist) and Biles II (a double twisting somersault). Gymnastics performance standards have been raised as a result of these advancements. Revolutionizing Difficulty: Biles has pushed the limits of what is technically feasible in gymnastics by incorporating daring and intricate components into her routines. Her efforts have raised the bar for the sport's level of difficulty and inventiveness.

Increasing the Complexity of Routines—High-Difficulty Combinations: The intricate arrangements of skills and components in Biles' routines push the boundaries of conventional knowledge. Her ability to deftly blend extremely challenging routines into her performances has raised the bar for gymnasts all throughout the world. Inspiring Technical Evolution: Her routines have encouraged other gymnasts to experiment with and incorporate novel methods, creating a culture where technical advancement is a constant in the sport.

Redefining the Parameters of Athletics Excellent Achievement Levels-Record-Breaking Achievements: Biles has broken numerous gymnastics records with her long list of successes, which includes multiple World Championship titles and Olympic medals. The criteria for success and greatness in the sport have been redefined by her achievements. Consistency and Dominance: She has set the standard for upcoming generations of competitors with her persistent dominance in contests, showcasing a level of excellence rarely seen in gymnastics.

Aiding in the Evaluation and Selection-Impact on the Code of Points**: Due to Biles' ground-breaking accomplishments, the gymnastics code of points has been modified to reflect the harder and more intricate nature of her routines. Her influence on scoring and judging has helped the sport's standards change over time. Shifting Scoring Expectations: Biles has changed the expectations for scoring by increasing the level of technical difficulty, which has motivated judges and gymnasts to concentrate on more intricate and precise execution.

Shifting How Women Athletes Are Seen Disturbing Stereotypes-Breaking Gender Norms: By dispelling myths about female athletes, Biles has shown that it is possible for women to reach astounding heights of strength, talent, and creativity. The way people view female athleticism has changed as a result of her achievements. Increasing Visibility: Her notoriety has increased awareness of women's sports and gymnasts, which has helped to level the playing field for equal acknowledgement of female athletes in the public and media.

Mary A.Clapp

Mental Health Advocacy-Promoting Well-Being: Biles' candidness regarding her battles with mental health has brought attention to how crucial mental health is for athletes. Her work has promoted a more encouraging atmosphere and broadened the debate around mental health in sports. Encouraging Open Dialogue: By being open about her experiences, Biles has lessened the stigma associated with talking about mental health and inspired other athletes to put their health first.

 Motivating Next Generations Young Athletes: A Role Model-Encouraging Aspiration: Young athletes find great motivation in Biles' accomplishments and tenacity. Her example inspires aspiring gymnasts to work hard and persistently towards their goals. Encouraging Self-Belief: Her success story shows that extraordinary things are achievable with hard work and self-belief, inspiring young people to strive for excellence and have faith in their own skills.

Progressive Possibilities—Building Pathways for Success: Biles's impact has aided in the development of new chances for gymnasts, such as greater money, support, and recognition. Her efforts aid in the expansion and advancement of the sport on all fronts. Fostering Talent: She has a significant influence on the up-and-coming gymnasts by mentoring and encouraging them, which helps to develop talent and guarantee the sport's continuous advancement.

Legacy and Implications for the Future Persistent Impact—Shaping Gymnastics' Future: By establishing new benchmarks and motivating upcoming generations of athletes, Biles' contributions will continue to define the sport of gymnastics. The changing methods and standards in the sport are ingrained in her legacy. Ongoing Inspiration: Simone Biles continues to inspire athletes, supporters, and fans worldwide even after her competitive career has ended.

Ongoing Protest-Advancing Important Issues : The sports community and beyond will continue to be impacted by Biles' persistent activism for gender equality and mental health. Her work makes the atmosphere for athletes more welcoming and encouraging.

Simone Biles' ground-breaking inventions, outstanding performances, and advocacy have permanently altered gymnastics. Her influence on the game has inspired new generations, disproved preconceptions, and redefined standards. Biles' career bears witness to both her amazing talent and her dedication to promoting essential principles in sports and gymnastics.

PERMANENT AFFECT ON SPORT AND SOCIETY

Simone Biles has had a profound impact on society at large as well as the sport of gymnastics, her reach going well beyond the gymnastics arena. Her contributions have changed people's opinions, sparked reform, and accelerated advancement in a number of spheres related to sports and public life.

Effect on Gymnastics Transforming Technical Guidelines- New Skills and Routines: Biles raised the bar for gymnastics' technical requirements by introducing cutting-edge skills and routines like the Biles and Biles II. Her efforts have changed the definition of difficulty and execution, raising the bar for gymnasts all around the world. Influencing Judging Criteria: Due to her performances, the gymnastics code of points and scoring criteria have been revised to reflect the difficulty and complexity of her routines, which have become more sophisticated. The progress of the sport has been aided by Biles' impact, which has changed the way gymnasts are viewed.

Creating New Reference Points-Record-Breaking Achievements: Biles has broken numerous world records and won multiple Olympic medals thanks to her incredible performances. Her accomplishment encourages gymnasts to strive for greater heights and sets a high bar for upcoming generations. Consistency and Excellence: Her unwavering domination and excellence have completely rewritten the rules for what constitutes competitive gymnastics success, emphasizing the value of perseverance and commitment.

Promoting Parity Among Sexes-Challenging Stereotypes: By proving that women are capable of remarkable feats of strength, skill, and inventiveness,

Biles has dispelled long-held misconceptions about female athletes. A more positive and accepting perception of female athleticism has resulted from her achievements. Increasing Visibility: Her notoriety has raised awareness of women's sports and female gymnastics, which has helped advance acceptance and encouragement for female athletes of all stripes.

The Impact of Society - Encouraging Awareness of Mental Health Breaking the Stigma: Biles' candidness about her battles with mental illness has contributed to the dismantling of the stigma associated with mental illness in athletes. Her advocacy has promoted open communication about mental health and created a more supportive atmosphere. Encouraging Self-Care: Her focus on the value of mental health and self-care has shaped the public's and athletes' perceptions of and priorities for mental health, which has led to a larger societal movement towards holistic health.

Motivating Next Generations-Role Model for Aspiring Athletes: Young athletes can draw a lot of inspiration from Biles' accomplishments and tenacity. Her narrative inspires everyone to follow their dreams with courage and tenacity, whether they are gymnasts or not. Empowering Young People: Her activism and success inspire young people to pursue excellence and believe in their own abilities, enabling them to overcome obstacles and have a positive influence.

Promoting Equality-Gender Equality in Sports: Biles has been a strong proponent of gender parity in sports, using her position to draw attention to pertinent concerns and lend support to projects in this area. Her initiatives support the continuous advancement of female athletes' recognition and equitable opportunity. Social Justice and Community Engagement: Biles' dedication to social justice and constructive change is demonstrated by her participation in charitable endeavors and neighborhood projects. Her donations promote a number of issues, such as youth development, health, and education.

 Legacy and Ongoing Impact Permanent Effect on Gymnastics - Shaping the Sport's Future: Gymnastics' standards, methods, and expectations will all be shaped by the legacy of gymnast Simone Biles. Her contributions will continue to be crucial to the growth and development of gymnastics. Inspiring New Talent: Biles' ideas and accomplishments will motivate upcoming gymnast generations to push limits and pursue perfection, guaranteeing her legacy in the sport.

Continuous Impact of Society- Cultural and Social Change: Biles' influence is felt in more general societal matters such as community support, mental health, and gender equality. Her support and good example advance ideals of resiliency, equality, and wellbeing while fostering continuous cultural and social transformation.

Continued Advocacy and Leadership: As long as Biles takes on leadership and advocacy responsibilities, her influence will probably keep promoting progress and motivating people in a variety of sectors. Gymnast Simone Biles has made a lasting impression on culture and gymnastics alike. Through her ground-breaking accomplishments, support of gender equality and mental health, and inspirational leadership, Biles has changed people's perspectives, raised the bar, and brought about good change. Future generations will be inspired by her enduring effect on the sport, which is a

255

testament to her remarkable legacy and continuous contributions to society at large.

Mary A.Clapp

CONCLUSION

Through her extraordinary accomplishments and efforts, Simone Biles has dramatically impacted gymnastics and influenced countless individuals. Her influence will continue to shape the sport and larger social conversations as we move forward. Here's a look at what's in store for Biles and the gymnastics community.

The prospects for Simone Biles Ongoing Effect in Gymnastics—Ongoing Contributions: As long as Biles keeps up her mentoring, coaching, and event-participating efforts, her impact in gymnastics is probably going to stay substantial. The way that upcoming generations view competition, technique, and training will be influenced by her legacy.

Potential for New Achievements: As Biles pursues her profession, more successes and milestones might be in store. Her unwavering dedication to innovation and quality raises the possibility that she will still break records and set new benchmarks.

Public Engagement and Advocacy Mental Health Advocacy: Biles will probably keep up her support of mental health, leveraging her position to spread knowledge, encouragement, and constructive change. Her initiative in this field will help create a more encouraging atmosphere for athletes and other people dealing with mental health issues.

Social and Community Initiatives: She will probably keep up her efforts to promote youth development, education, and other causes that are near and dear to her heart as part of her ongoing dedication to philanthropy and community involvement.

Gymnastics's Prospects Changing Procedures and Standards Influence on the Sport: Biles's influence will continue to shape the technical requirements and expectations in gymnastics. Her inventions have changed the way routines are created and assessed by setting new standards for performance and complexity.

Inspiration for Innovation: Biles' ground-breaking routines and methods will serve as an inspiration for upcoming gymnasts, spurring continuous innovation and advancement in the sport. Her influence will motivate upcoming generations of athletes to strive for greater success.

 A Greater Aim for Equality and Well-Being Integration of Mental Health: Biles's activism has brought attention to the significance of mental health in athletics. It is anticipated that attention to athlete well-being will increase, with a greater focus on fostering supportive settings and attending to mental health concerns.

Gender Equality Advancements: Thanks to Biles' advocacy and example, the movement towards more gender equality in sports will continue to gain traction. Her work will help female athletes get more attention, encouragement, and opportunity.

Mary A.Clapp

 Legacy and Persistent Impact Persistent
Motivation—Role Model for Future Generations: Biles
will continue to motivate young people and athletes with
her legacy as a role model. Her accomplishments and
fortitude teach us important lessons about tenacity,
excellence, and self-belief.

Cultural Impact: Gymnastics' perception and value
inside the sport as well as in larger social contexts will
be shaped by Biles' career for years to come.

Ongoing Collaboration—Leadership and Mentorship:
Biles's guidance and leadership will be vital in
determining the direction gymnastics takes as she
moves into new positions. Her mentoring will support the
development of the upcoming generation of gymnasts
and further the sport's continuous advancement.

Public Influence: Biles will continue to be a well-known
public figure who uses her position to promote crucial
causes and spur constructive change. Her influence on
gymnastics and society will increase If she stays
involved. Simone Biles's ground-breaking
accomplishments, advocacy, and inspirational

Mary A.Clapp

leadership have made a lasting impact on gymnastics
and society.

Her impact will continue to alter the sport and bring
about significant change as we look to the future. Future
generations will be inspired by Biles' legacy of brilliance,
tenacity, and advocacy, which will propel gymnastics
and other sports forward. Her influence will likely last for
many years to come, thanks to her continued
involvement and efforts.